Proceedings and Collections
Anti-cancer, anti-cancer metastasis research

THE NARRATE OF INNOVATION THEORIES

and

METHODS OF CANCER TREATMENT VOLUME 3

Reform • Innovation • Development

The promising prospects of Immunomodulating drugs

Authors: Bin Wu, Lily Xu
Editors: Bin Wu, Lily Xu,
Translators: Bin Wu, Lily Xu

authorHOUSE

AuthorHouse™
1663 Liberty Drive
Bloomington, IN 47403
www.authorhouse.com
Phone: 833-262-8899

Published by AuthorHouse 09/13/2021

ISBN: 978-1-6655-3698-1 (sc)
ISBN: 978-1-6655-3697-4 (e)

Library of Congress Control Number: 2021913205

Print information available on the last page.

This book is printed on acid-free paper.

The human body is a hero.
All healing of the human body is an innate self healing
and is an inherent biological process.
Our health is controlled by our hands.
We are the drivers for our health.

The doctors are at their best with modifying, regulating, controlling the circumstances, the conditions under which we live, such as what type of diet, how much rest we have, how mch food we take, how much sleep we have, how much exercise we have, how much worry not justified, how much anxiety not justified.

It is very important in our lifes to stay in the present time, the present is a gift. This is the way we should think of and this is the way we should live.

The main purpose for us to be healthy, it is that where we have the state of functional excellence which allow us to get the best mentally and physically and spiritually for ourselves (our organisum or our bodies).

The cancer cure should be through regulation and controlling rather than killing

In this book, I summary the new things and our past work together in the detail, <u>especially emphazie the medications for cancer treatment.</u>

Life is precious and let us prevent from cancer and other diseases.

Let us learn the things through hard work and others wisdom.

THE IMPORTANT CONCEPT OF CANCER TREATMENT

The cancer cure should be through regulation and control rather than killing.

Healing should be through regulation and control rather than killing.

The last step in curing cancer is to mobilize the reappearance of the host's control, rather than destroy the last cancer cells.

Cancer prevention is the same important as cancer treatment.

In another word, keeping our bodied healthy immune function is essential for completely curing cancer.

For the aboving concepts, there are some experiments to support them as the followings in brief:

From the father of medicine Hippocrates, "Everyone has a physician inside him or her; we just have to help it in its work. The natural healing force within each one of us is the greatest force in getting well. The next questions:

How can we wake up widely our inside physician?

Now along the technological rapid development, our human being works very hard to search for the good ways to live longer and to keep diseases free such as fasting, medication, meditation etc.

From Chinese book **"Huang Di Nei Jing"**, it is also said, *"the disease is not the inherent part of human body, which can be gained and also can be removed. If it can not be removed, it is because the method is not found.*

This means, the health is our normal state. If any disease happens to us, we should or could find the correct way to remove it. Our inherent part is health.

From Shong Han Theory, it is said, "*losing grain can cure the diseases*".

With thousand years people work hard to search for the ways for curing the diseases.

Where is the way for cancer theory?
How can it make cancer free from us?
How can we remove the cancer fear from us?

During our experiments, we surprisely found that cancer can disappear by their own or even if the cancer cells are injected into the body, the cancer will not grow at all.

Here some example of our experiments which were done as the following in brief, the detail and more experiment will be explained in detail in this book chapters:

1. From experimental studies, the process of cancer cell metastasis in the lymphatic tract was observed:

A. After transplanting 1×10^6 cancer cells under the skin of the inner side of the mouse paw pads, the animals were sacrificed at different times for local lymph node histological observation.

One hour after the transplantation of tumor cells, a single cancer cell was found in the marginal sinus of the cochineal lymph node, but no mitotic phase was seen;

After 3 hours, there are 3-5 groups of tumor cells in the marginal sinus of the cochineal lymph node, and mitotic phases can be seen;

After 5 hours, there are piles of cancer cells in the marginal sinus of the rouge lymph node, and some tumor cells have entered the middle sinus.

Twenty-four hours later, metastases had formed in the rouge lymph nodes. Scattered cancer cells were found in the middle sinus.

After 3-5 days, the popliteal lymph nodes have been occupied by metastatic tumor cells, and tumor cells and metastatic lesions were found in the second and third lymph nodes near the iliac artery and renal hilum.

Generally, metastases can be found in multiple lymph nodes after 3 days. Some cancer cells (such as Ehrlich's ascites carcinoma) form metastases only 5 days, and the metastases of rouge fossa lymph nodes can undergo degeneration and necrosis, and lymph node immune cells proliferate.

However, after 10 days, no cancer cells were found in the lymph nodes, and they were eventually destroyed by the host cells and disappeared.

The above experimental results suggest:

5 days after Ehrlich ascites cancer cells form metastases, the rouge lymph nodes may **undergo degeneration and necrosis**.

It indicates that the lymph node itself is a peripheral immune organ, which should be monitored and swallowed by cancer cells.

After 10 days, no cancer cells were found in the lymph nodes, which were obviously eliminated by the host's immune cells.

It is suggested that the treatment of anti-cancer metastasis can use the anti-cancer system and anti-cancer factors to protect and activate the host to destroy the invading cancer cells. The immune defense in the body can remove the cancer cells completely.

B. *Carry out experimental research on tumors and create cancer-bearing animal models*

A sterile tumor specimen was removed from the clinical operating table, and it was transplanted into experimental animals after 0.5h of warm ischemia. It was done more than 100 times (400 animals) without success. There was no any single animal which grew cancer yet.

However, when the thymus was first removed and then the cancer cells were transplanted in some mice, the cancer cells grew in the mice, which means after the removal of the main immune organ Thymus, it can promote the cancer cell growth. And this experiment was successful in the 210 animals.

Some injections of cortisone can reduce the immunity of mice and it can also promote the cancer cell growth so that the cancer cells can be transplanted successfully to the mice.

5 days after the thymus is cut and the cancer cells were transplanted, the large soybean nodules can grow after 5-6 days, and they grew to a large tumor of the thumb in 10-21 days.

Transplanted cancer can survive for 3-4 weeks, but it cannot be passed down to generations.

1. *Through this study, it is found that removal of the thymus can create a cancer-bearing animal model, and injection of cortisone can also help create a cancer-bearing animal model.*

2. *Research conclusions prove that the occurrence and development of cancer are related to the host's body immunity, and have a very obvious relationship with immune organs and immune organ tissue functions.*

3. *The results of this study confirmed that the immune organ thymus (Thymus, Th) and immune function have an extremely definite relationship with the occurrence and development of cancer.*

If the host Thymus is removed, it may be made into a cancer-bearing animal model, and if it is not removed, it cannot be a cancer-bearing animal model.

Injecting immunosuppressive drugs to reduce host immunity function will help create cancer-bearing animal models. Without injections of immuno-lowering drugs, cancer-bearing animal models cannot be created.

This result shows that immune organs and immunity are negatively correlated with cancer cell growth (during the cancer transplantation experiment and cancer implanation experiment) into solid cancer.

With immunodeficiency or reduced immunity, cancer cells of transplantation can implant and grow tumors without being swallowed or destroyed or damaged by the host's immune cells.

C. **From the animal experiments, cancer cells S_{180} 1×10^6 were injected into** Kuanming mouse through the tail vein, which were eliminated by 99% after 24-36 hours, and only less than 0.1 of cancer cells can be survived and can be grown and form the metastasis.

Who destroyed these 99% cancer cells?

It suggested that some of cancer cells were destroyed by the uncomfortable environment or the crash force or obstracting in the circulation of blood, however the most of the cancer cells after entering into the blood circulation mainly be destroyed by the host immune defences system such as the immune cells.

Hence, it should protect the host immune sysmentand should activate the host immune system function during treating the cancer and should not strike the host immune system and should not decreasethe host immune defense function.

In this book, there are many ways which are provided to protect the host immune functions.

In brief, healing is a biological process and is innate. Our body is the hero. There is no such things as chemicals, drugs, food and other ingredient that will take place of the living process of life.

All healing is self healing. Healing is not something that somebody else does to you. Healing is something you do for yourself.

The miracle is the living process and is it-self but what the doctor can do is the doctor can make decision about lifestyle which can enhance the person life or destroy the person life.

The choice or general speaking is yours and you have to make these decisions.

This is a book of the summary and reflection of the part of the past work for the cancer theorepy.

The extremely important concepts of cancer prevention:

1. **_Cancer is a disease that can be prevented_** because now sinscien already proved that more than 90% of cancer occurrence are related to the environmental factors such as air, water, food, soil, and the social environment, etc.
2. Cancer is a diseae that threatens the human life so that the human **_should prevent and treat cancer_**; meanwhile it should realize that cancer can be prevented and cured; also it is very important to realize **_that cancer prevention should be put on the same attention and the same level at the same time_** in order to stop and to eliminate the cancer occurrence at its source and before cancer happens.
3. **_It should do three early things: the early discovery, the early diagnosis, the early treatment. Cancer can be cured_**.

CONTENTS

Part V

The Experimental Research

Part VI

**The case list & some typical cases of XZ-C immune regulation and
control anti-cancer Chinese medicine treatment of cancer**

TO ALL MY READERS

First, I deeply appreciate you for taking your precious time to open this book about the wellness of human beings.

Why do cancer and metastasis happen?
How should we treat it?
Can it be reversed by our bodies?
Can cancer be reversed and, if so, how?

During our experiments, some of the cancer in the rats disappeared after the cancer cells already moved to lymph nodes on the day of 8. When we injected cancer cells into mice and the lymph nodes had necrosis, eventually, the cancer disappeared.

All of these proved that our bodies had the ability to eliminate the cancer cells during our repeated experiments.

How can we help our bodies activate or enhance these abilities to remove cancer cells?
How can our body's physician be woken up to remove all cancer cells?

Technology has been dramatically developed, and many mysteries in the past have been clearly explained by scientific evidence. Many chronic diseases such as heart disease, cancer, metabolic diseases, and diabetics can be prevented and cured.

Cancer prevention is as important as the cancer treatment (it must be emphasized that prevention and treatment need the same attention and the same lever at the same time).

This book mainly emphasizes the medications which we use for treating cancer patients, especially the immunotherapy medications (the drugs' mechanism, the experiments, and the clinical verifications, etc).

In this book, many basic and clinical experiments in the lab proved and provided that cancer treatment should be through controlling it and should regulate the recovery of the body's ability of controlling the cancer, not through killing the final cancer cell. These experiments proved many of the new and important theories, such as:

The leading or guiding ideas of the new cancer model are:

Regulation and signal transmission between cells in cancer patients are disrupted rather than lost; the carcinogenesis is considered to be a *<u>continuum with the possibility of reversal.</u>*

Or it is considered that carcinogenesis is a continuum with the **possibility of reversal.**

<u>**Our body is constantly changing all the time and today's you is different from tomorrow's you.**</u>

Let us gather our knowledge:

1. *When I reviewed Greek medicine, the words from the father of medicine, Hippocrates gave me great relevance about our health:*

    <u>"Everyone has a physician inside him or her; we just have to help it in its work. The natural healing force within each one of us is the greatest force in getting well. Our food should be our medicine. Our medicine should be our food. But to eat when you are sick is to feed your sickness."</u>

    - Hippocrates

This means our body has infinite healing wisdom.

<u>How can we wake up completely this inner physician or search out this inside physician to get complete recovery?</u>

In this book, we have written down some of this wisdom in detail, with some of the experiments in medication (the evidence), methods for cancer treatment, etc., which it can benefit our human health.

<u>**In this book, there are many medications which were tested and verified, and they had excellent effects on cancer patients.**</u>

Of course, there are many other ways such as fasting, exercise, meditation, etc.

2. *Technology has rapidly developed.*

Many things which we once thought of as impossible have now been achieved.

The understanding of life, such as physiology, pathogenetic pathophysiology, genetics, etc. grows fast as new technology and science develops rapidly after the knowledge and findings of humans increase.

Many mysteries of the living body have been explained and verified or confirmed by facts, such as:

1) Some cardiovascular diseases can be reversed, and *nitric oxide*, especially the **endothelium cell** is important for the vascular system to function well (1).

It was found that good circulation is the key for our health, such as cancer metastasis and for our immune system (. As Dr. William Osler said: we are as old as our arteries.

2) Hyperinsulinemia (insulin resistance) and high carbohydrates are related to many diseases, such as diabetes (diabetes can be reversed completely), to the fibroid and to prostate diseases (2, 3, 4)

3) Our body can recycle to keep healthy, which is good for aging and many other diseases. It also has proven the concepts for many disease treatments, for a variety of diseases, which comes from the Nobel Prize in Physiology or Medicine 2016, awarded to Yoshinori Ohsumi "for his discoveries of mechanisms for autophagy." The concept gave evidence for fasting therapy for many diseases, such as aging, diabetics, cancer, and others more.

4) Our endocrine system is extremely important and related to many cancers and other diseases, such as estrogen (it is clear to relate this with breast cancer and other cancers, but especially those found in women), testosterone (it is one of the factors which is related to prostate cancer growth), *insulin (which is related to many conditions of the body)*, etc.

The human being is evolving and is now a hormonally modified human being. It is very important to keep the hormone balance between catabolism and anabolism, mainly by insulin (from the pancreas) and other hormones.

Our daily habits change our hormone levels so that if we change our habits, we can control our hormone balance to control our health situation. We will become the drivers for our health.

In addition, Hippocrates, the father of Western **medicine**, believed **fasting** enabled the body to heal itself. (He believed in the infinite healing wisdom inside human beings).

Paracelsus, another great healer in the Western tradition, wrote 500 years ago that "**fasting** is the greatest remedy, the physician within."

In brief, lifestyle changes are extremely important for our health, our aging, and our mind. This discipline is extremely important to keep good health.

3. *In Chinese <<Huangdi neijing>>, there were:*

The disease is not the thing belonging to our bodies, which can come and can be removed. If the disease cannot be removed, it is because the correct methods have not been found.

Persistence, persistence, and persistence!

During the time of COVID-19, I have stayed at home reviewing many medical textbooks about anatomy, biochemistry, immunology as well as clinical and experimental research data. One lecture I listened to repeatedly was given by a surgeon. One phrase that stuck out to me was, "Perhaps brains are important, but nothing and nothing is as important as persistence, persistence, and persistence.

"The road of science is not smooth, and similarly, neither is the road of life. After a long, challenging, and tearing road, this is finally here now."

How is this book new and what is it about?

This book focuses on cancer prevention and treatment, specifically on immune pharmacy.

We must accept the factors:

Technology is developing dramatically; the wonders of modern technology make many mysteries clear and clinical data has shown that many diseases can be cured and prevented by lifestyle changes and by our inside systems.

However, cancer is still a dangerous disease that threatens many people's wellbeing.

How can we help control these diseases?

What is the road that can cure and prevent these diseases?

This book will discuss a new way of controlling and preventing cancer. I hope you enjoy reading.

References:

(1) Prevent and Reverse Heart Disease: The Revolutionary, Scientifically Proven, Nutrition-Based Cure, by Caldwell B. Esselstyn Jr. Publisher : Avery; 1st edition (January 31, 2008)

(2) Hyperinsulinemia: An Early Indicator of Metabolic Dysfunction, Dylan D Thomas, Barbara E Corkey, Nawfal W Istfan, Caroline M Apovian.
Journal of the Endocrine Society, Volume 3, Issue 9, September 2019, Pages 1727–1747, https://doi.org/10.1210/js.2019-00065

(3) Diet-Induced Hyperinsulinemia as a Key Factor in the Etiology of Both Benign Prostatic Hyperplasia and Essential Hypertension?
Wolfgang Kopp, Mariatrosterstrasse 41, 8043 Graz, Austria.
Nutr Metab Insights. 2018; 11: 1178638818773072. Published online 2018 May 8. doi: 10.1177/1178638818773072 PMCID: PMC6238249 PMID: 30455570

(4) Uterine Leiomyomata in Relation to Insulin-Like Growth Factor-I, Insulin, and Diabetes.
Donna Day Baird,1 Greg Travlos,2 Ralph Wilson,2 David B Dunson,3 Michael C Hill,4 Aimee A D'Aloisio,1 Stephanie J London,1 and Joel M Schectman5
Published in final edited form as: Epidemiology. 2009 Jul; 20(4): 604–610. PMC2856640 PMID: 19305350

(5) International narcotics control board for 2009. New York: United Nations, 2010). Canadian Gazette. Controlled Drugs and Substances Ac

(6) The book<< new concept and new ways of treatment of cancer metastasis>>. Xu Ze, etc. Pressed in 2016 by authorhouse Inc. U.SA

Bin Wu, Lily Xu
04-27-21, in Timonium, Maryland USA

ABOUT THE AUTHOR 1

**A brief introduction to the first author
and the main translator and the editor**

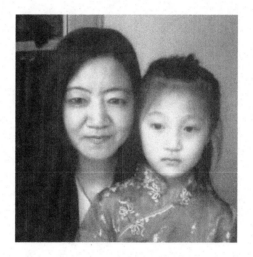

Bin Wu, MD, Ph.D., graduated from College of Yunyang of Tongji University of Medical Sciences for her MD degree; Studied her Master degree and her Ph. D degree in Sun Yat-Sen University of Medical Sciences. After she received her Ph.D., she worked as a Post-doctoral fellow in the Johns Hopkins Medical School and University of Maryland Medical School. She passed all of her USMLE tests and is going to do her residency training in America. She dedicated herself to oncology clinical and research. Her goal is to conquer cancer, which she believes this great contribution to our health. She has a daughter, named Lily Xu who gives great help with writing and editing and drawing all of the pictures in the books.

ABOUT THE AUTHOR 2

**A Brief introduction to the second author and
the editor and my only trustful advisor**

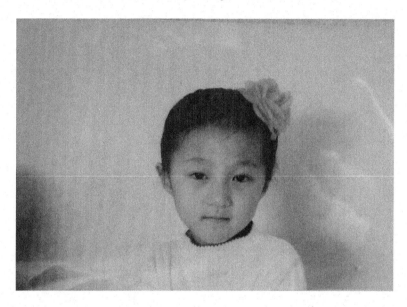

Lily Xu was born on November 17th 2006 and is in Advanced Biology Class in the high school since 2020. In 2020, she won the Robot designing model in Maryland and Math Model in Baltimore County in Maryland and she is in the Baltimore country honor banding. She helps with this book edition and others. She had an art presented in the Walter Art Museum in Baltimore at the age of 6; she got the fourth place trophy in the ES Double Digits or 24 and 24 games in the Baltimore County in Maryland; she got the first trophy in the BCPS STEM FAIR PHYSICS in Baltimore County; when she was in the sixth grade, she passed the advanced Math for 7th grade(which means the 8th grade math) test and moved the 8th grade math class and now she takes high school Math class; she loves the reading and the writing and she finished many seires of books and in 2019 summary she start to do volunteer job in the publish libarary. She got $9000 scholarship award for the Peabody music program in the Johns Hopkins University. She edits all of my books for the publishing and drew all of the pictures in this book. In 2018 and 2019 she was chosen into Baltimore county Middle school Honor Band. In 2018 the robotic team which she attended for years got designing-award from the Baltimore county so that this robotic team came to Maryland State for the Robotic contest in 2019. On January 19th, 2019 she got the Robotic designing award in Maryland. She edits all of my books for the publishing and drew all of the pictures in the book. In 2019 she was chosen by Baltimore County for one duel and one ensemble to play Clarion. Now she is in the nineth grade for her high school and while she was chosen to attend of Maryland state debate team in March 2021. She loves study and challenge and has execellent judgement. In 2021, she already won four medals for the different contests.

PREFACE

This monographs is not only written with a pen, *but also made with real and hard work or done with actually working or performing.*

The contents of these monographs all come from clinical practice experience and lessons, review, reflection, and **practice produces the reality and practice leads to know the truth**.

The contents of these monographs are all derived from the experimental research results of their own laboratories, and **the experiments produced results or achievement.**

The content of these monographs is a true record of scientific thinking and scientific practice from experiment to clinical, and then from clinical to experimental. The summary of experimental research and clinical verification data has risen to the essence of theory; meanwhile the new discoveries, new understandings, and new theories have been proposed. **All of these innovative theories of clinical practicability can be used to guide clinical treatment**.

All should be converted to clinical applications through translational medicine to guide clinical treatment and benefit patients.

The contents of these monographs:

They are all their own more than half a century of therapeutic practice experience and 30 years of experimental research materials. They are summarized, organized, and compiled into this book. The scientific research results and scientific and technological innovation series **are all their own materials, and some of them are international firsts. All of them are the original innovation. Some are internationally advanced and independent innovations, all with independent intellectual property rights.**

The content of this series of monographs:

Fully or completely is in line with or corresponds to the content of translational medicine.

Our 28-year scientific research route has been from clinical to experimental, clinical and experimental, and returns to the clinical to solve clinical practical problems. Our research model is completely in line with or matches this new medical research model.

Translational or transformation Medicine

Transformation Medicine recently develops rapidly and vigorously internationally.

This new medical research model advocates patient-centered, discovering and asking questions from clinical work, conducting in-depth basic research, and then quickly turning basic research results into clinical applications to improve the overall level of medical care and ultimately benefit patients.

Academician Chen Zhu, the former minister of the Ministry of Health, has analyzed the connotation of translational medicine:

First, translational medicine is a science that passes **through a two-way channel from laboratory to clinic and from clinical to laboratory for In-depth understanding the mechanisms of the occurrence and development of diseases and mechanisms of health protection promotion, and exploring new prevention and control strategies.**

Second, we **must transform scientific research results into clinical, public health, practical, interventional methods, technologies, and programs for their popularization.**

The World Health Organization proposes that medicine in the 21st century should not continue to use disease as the main research field, but should take human health as the main research direction.

Academician Chen Zhu pointed out:

The health service model should be transformed. It is necessary to shift from treatment-oriented in the late stage of serious diseases to prevention-oriented, and move the gate forward and sink the center of gravity. Strengthening research

in preventive medicine is a major issue in my country and the transformation of the global medical model.

The focus of my country's translational or transformation medicine research, the modernization and internationalization of Chinese medicine and Chinese medication is one of the key contents of my country's translational medicine research.

ACKNOWLEDGEMENTS

When I was close to finish this book, I recalled my parents dramatically because I realized their words and behaviour and spirit are so useful for me to live well. I looked at my parents and my childhood pictures and many beautiful momery showed up. I learned things from my parents. Now I realize that my father was such an excellent person on the healthy skills and the wisest doctor in my mind. He realized that the lifestyle of an individual is such an important thing for preventing and curing a disease. I learn to have a strong will.

If they were still alive, I would understand more medicine and do more things for others because I would get more things from their experience.

I thank my parents to enlighten me about the medicine since I started to understand things. My parents want me to do more contribution our societies.

When I was at the very young age, my father told me **how the bone morrow is important**. At that time, I didn't understand anything about immune system. My mother always told me something such **as garlic, ginger** function and why we eat them while I watched her cooked the dishes.

I thank my parents for trying very hard to lead me like to become a medical professional because both of them really loved what they dedicate and they wanted me to follow their footsteps. Both them let me come to the operation room to shadow them even far before I went to medical school. My father was excellent on many medical things. I miss my parents.

In addition, I **thank for Lily Xu who helps me editing all of my work and always give me the great and crystal idea and suggestion. She told me that the grammar should be paid attention to.** Thank for she studied hard by her own so that I can concentrate on this book.

Second, this book is for all of people who concern human being health.

We are deep grateful to all of people who like our new ways to improve our human being health. I appreciate to anyone who encourages me to continue working on my career. I thank for any good word which is encouraging me.

My daughter Lily Xu gives me many smart and creative ideas while we were finishing this book. **The characteristics of she loves the challenge** and her judgment always encourages me to continue working hard to move on. I learn the new things from her daily. I have to admit she is really smart on thinking things.

I would like to express our sincere gratitude to the following:

1. All of Authorhouse staffs

2. Dr. Xu Ze and other workers who were involved in cancer patient care.

3. Mrs. Bo Wu's family and Mrs. Tao Wu's famly

4. I deeply thank my only daughter Lily Xu, for her help with me and for her wisdom, for <u>her understanding me</u> and for <u>her update knowledge and for her loving learning</u>.

Bin Wu, M.D., Ph.D
04-29-2021 in Timonium, Maryland in USA

This book is the summary and collections of the part of the past work.

1. **The important concept <u>*of cancer treatment*</u>:**

   <u>**The cancer cure should be through regulation and control rather than killing.**</u>

   Healing should be through regulation and control rather than killing.

   The last step in curing cancer is to mobilize the reappearance of the host's control, rather than destroy the last cancer cells.

   <u>*In another word, keeping our bodied healthy immune function is essential for completely curing cancer.*</u>

2. **The important concept *of cancer prevention*:**

Cancer prevention is the same importance as cancer treatment. It should put on the same attention and the same level at the same time. It is very important to do three early things: the early discovery, the early diagnosis, the early treatment so that cure can be cured.

For the aboving concepts, we have some experients to support them in the following book content in the details.

FOREWORD

Gratifying or Improving prospects for immunomodulatory drugs

No matter how complicated the mechanism behind cancer is, the body's immune suppression is the key to cancer progression.

Removal of immunosuppressive factors and restoration of system cells' recognition of cancer cells <u>can effectively defeat or resist cancer</u>. More and more research evidence shows that by regulating the body's immune system, it is possible to achieve the purpose of controlling cancer. The treatment of tumors by activating the body's anti-tumor immune system is currently an exciting area for researchers. The next major breakthrough in cancer is likely to come from this.

<u>In order to discuss the etiology, pathogenesis, and pathophysiology of cancer, we conducted a series of animal experimental studies. From the analysis of experimental results, we have obtained the new discoveries and new enlightenments:</u>

<u>Atrophy of the thymus and low or decreasing immune function are one of the causes and pathogenesis of cancer. Therefore, Professor Xu Ze proposed at the international conference that one of the causes and pathogenesis of cancer may be atrophy of the thymus and impaired function of the central immune organs, immune function decreasing, immune surveillance ability reducing and immune escape.</u>

As a result of laboratory experiments, it was found that:

The thymus of cancer-bearing mice showed progressive atrophy. The function of the central immune organ is impaired, the immune function is reduced, and the immune surveillance is low, *<u>so the treatment principle must be to prevent the thymus from progressive atrophy, to promote thymus hyperplasia, to protect the bone marrow hematopoietic function and to improve immune surveillance, which provides a theoretical basis and experimental basis for treatment of cancer with immune regulation and control.</u>*

Based on the enlightenment of the above experimental results on cancer etiology and pathogenesis, the new concepts and methods of XZ-C immunomodulatory therapy are proposed.

After 16 years of clinical examination and observation of more than 12,000 middle-stage and advanced-stage cancer patients in the oncology clinic, *__it has been confirmed that the treatment principle of Thymus protection and enhancing immune function is reasonable and the efficacy is satisfactory.__*

__The application of immunomodulatory Chinese medicine has achieved good results, improved the quality of life, and significantly prolonged the survival period.__

__The XZ-C (XU ZE-China) immunomodulation method__ was first proposed by Professor Xu Ze in his book "New Concepts and Methods of Cancer Metastasis Treatment" in 2006.

He believes that **under normal circumstances, the cancer and the body's defenses are in a dynamic balance, and the occurrence of cancer is caused by the imbalance of the dynamic balance**. If the disordered state is adjusted to a normal level, the growth of cancer can be controlled and resolved, or if it is to adjust the disordered state to a normal level, it can control the growth of cancer and make cancer fade.

__As we all know, the occurrence, development and prognosis of cancer are determined by the comparison of two factors, that is, the biological characteristics of cancer cells and the host body's own defense ability to restrict and defend against cancer cells. If the two are balanced, the cancer can be controlled; if the two are out of balance, the cancer will develop.__

__Under normal circumstances, the host's body itself has certain restrictions on cancer cells, but when the host's body is suffering from cancer, these restrictions and defense capabilities are inhibited and damaged to varying degrees, resulting in cancer cells losing immune surveillance and cancer cell immune escape so that cancer cells can further develop and metastasize.__

Through the above 4 years of basic experimental research on the mechanism of recurrence and metastasis. After another 3 years of the tumor-inhibiting test in cancer-bearing mice from the internal experiment of natural medicine and herbal medicine. A batch of Chinese medicines with good tumor suppression rate were selected from Chinese herbal medicines to form XZ-C $_{1-10}$ anti-cancer immune-modulating Chinese medicine.

Part V

The Experimental Research

The experimental study on the etiology, pathogenesis and pathophysiology of cancer

CONTENTS

1

Preamble

The experimental surgery is extremely important in the development of medicine. It is the key to opening the restricted medical zone or the forbidden area of medicine.

<u>The prevention and treatment methods</u> of many diseases are applied to the clinic only after many animal experimental studies have achieved or obtained stability results, which it is to promote the development of the medical industry or career and of medical undertaking.

Experimental research and basic research are very important.

Without breakthroughs in experimental research and basic research, it is difficult to improve clinical efficacy, and it is difficult to come up with new understandings, new concepts, and new theoretical insights.

The laboratory is a key condition for the development of science and technological innovation.

I deeply understand the importance of laboratories. I am the first batch or group of college students who took the college entrance examination after liberation. I have no refresher course or have not studied abroad. However, I have achieved many international level results. **The key is that I have a good laboratory.**

<u>In the 1960s</u>, I participated in the open heart surgery laboratory with <u>cardiopulmonary bypass</u>.

In the 1980s, I established *<u>a cirrhotic ascites laboratory.</u>*

I established *<u>the Experimental Surgery Research Institute in the 1990s, with a focus on conquering cancer or with the main attack direction as conquering cancer.</u>*

My animal laboratory has good equipment conditions. It has animal experiments on mice, rats, guinea pigs, rabbits, dogs, monkeys, etc. It has a good sterilization or disinfection operating room, which can perform various major operations on the chest and abdomen, and has the animal observation room after surgery, which is able to achieve results or conclusions of various designs and ideas through experimental operations.

__Therefore, the laboratory is a key condition, and the key is to build a well-equipped laboratory. If there is no laboratory to pass through the experiment, it can only design and imagine, and it cannot become a fact.__

"Oncology" is currently the most backward subject in various medical disciplines.

Because the etiology, pathogenesis, and pathophysiology of oncology are not clearly understood, the oncology subject is still a scientific virgin land for scientific research, and it needs a lot of basic scientific research..

Although many countries have invested a lot of money in the treatment of cancer patients, although the three traditional treatment methods have been used for nearly a hundred years, the death rate of cancer is still the first cause of death in China's urban and rural residents.

The main reasons are as follows:

1) *The cause of cancer is not yet fully understood; people still lack sufficient understanding of the pathogenesis and the mechanism of cancer cell metastasis.*

2) *There is still insufficient understanding of the complicated biological behavior and pathophysiology of cancer.*

To carry out basic cancer research, anti-cancer metastasis, and recurrence, *basic research on cancer-bearing animal models* must be conducted.

Nude mice should be used to establish various cancer metastasis animal models to study the law and mechanism of cancer metastasis (the author's laboratory uses purebred Kunming mice are used as cancer-bearing animal models, about 10,000 times), because without breakthroughs in basic research, it is difficult to improve the clinical efficacy.

No matter how complicated the mechanism behind cancer is, immune suppression is the key to cancer progression.

Removing immunosuppressive factors and restoring the recognition of cancer cells by system cells can effectively defend against cancer.

More and more research evidences show that by regulating the body's immune system, it is possible to achieve the goal of cancer control.

The treatment of tumors by activating the body's anti-tumor immune system is an area that currently excites researchers, and the next major breakthrough in cancer is likely to come from this.

In order to explore the cause, pathogenesis, and pathophysiology of cancer, we conducted a series of animal experimental studies. From the analysis of experimental results, we obtained the new discoveries and new enlightenments:

Thymus atrophy and weakened immune function are one of the causes and pathogenesis of cancer.

Therefore, Professor Xu Ze proposed at an international conference that one of the causes and pathogenesis of cancer may be atrophy of the thymus, impaired central immune organ function, weakened immune function, decreased immune surveillance ability and immune escape.

The central immune organ has the closest relationship with tumor immunity. The thymus is the central immune organ and the place where T cells develop and mature. It plays a decisive role *in cellular immunity and even the entire immune regulation.*

As a result of laboratory experimental research it was found:

The thymus glands of cancer-bearing mice showed progressive atrophy, the central immune organ function was impaired, the immune function decreased, and immune surveillance was low.

Therefore, the treatment principle must be to prevent the progressive atrophy of the thymus, promote thymic hyperplasia, protect the bone marrow hematopoietic function, improve immune surveillance, and provide a theoretical basis and experimental basis for immune regulation and control treatment of cancer.

Based on the enlightenment from the above experimental research results on the etiology and pathogenesis of cancer, a new concept and new method of XZ-C immunomodulatory therapy is proposed.

After 16 years of clinical observation and observation of more than 12,000 cases of intermediate and advanced cancer patients in the oncology clinic, ***it is proved that the treatment principle of Thymus protection and immune function promotion is reasonable and the curative effect is satisfactory.***

The application of immune control Chinese medicine has achieved good results, improved the quality of life, and significantly extended the survival period.

XZ-C (XU ZE China) immunomodulation method was first proposed by Professor Xu Ze in his book "New Concepts and New Methods of Cancer Metastasis Treatment" in 2006.

He believes that under normal circumstances, there is a dynamic balance between cancer and the body's defenses, and the occurrence of cancer is caused by imbalance in dynamic balance. If the disordered state is adjusted to a normal level, the growth of the cancer can be controlled and it can be eliminated.

As we all know, the occurrence, development and prognosis of cancer are determined by the comparison of two factors, namely, the biological characteristics of cancer cells and the host body's ability to restrict and defend against cancer cells. If the two are balanced, cancer can be controlled.

If the two are out of balance, cancer develops.

Under normal circumstances, the host's body itself has a certain ability to restrict cancer cells, but when suffering from cancer, these restrictive defense capabilities are inhibited and damaged to varying degrees, resulting in cancer cells losing immune surveillance and cancer cell immune escape, which make the cancer cells further develop and metastasize.

Through the above 4 years of basic experimental research to explore the mechanism of recurrence and metastasis and after three years of the experiments for tumor suppression test in cancer-bearing mice for natural medicines and Chinese herbal medicines, a batch of Chinese medicines with good tumor inhibition rates were screened out from Chinese herbal medicines to form $XZ-C_{1-10}$ anti-cancer immune regulation and control chinese medication.

In the past 7 years, a series of clinical basic experimental research and basic problems exploration on more than 6,000 tumor-bearing animal models. The anti-tumor experiment screening of 200 kinds of Chinese herbal medicines in tumor-bearing animal models was done by several graduate students of mine:

1. *"Experimental study on the effect of spleen on tumor growth and the anti-cancer effect of Jianpi Yiqi Decoction" completed by Master Zhu Siping;*

2. *"Experimental study on the treatment of malignant tumors by adoptive immune reconstruction combined with transplantation of fetal liver, spleen and thymocytes" was completed by Dr. Shaomin Zou;*

3. *"Experimental study on the anti-tumor effect of Fuzheng Guben on S180-bearing mice" was completed by Master Li Zhengxun;*

4. *"Experimental study on the inhibitory effect of Huanglateng Acetate Acetate Extract (TG) on tumor neovascularization in mice", completed by Master Liu Liling.*

The topics for master and doctoral students are all subtopics of our general topic, all of which are clinical basic problems that are closely integrated with clinical practice. They have carried out and completed a large number of painstaking and meticulous experimental research work. The bitter, round-the-clock experimental research work has made a significant contribution to the development of the experimental oncology medicine for **cancer prevention and anti-cancer.**

2

The new discoveries from the experimental tumor research on anti-cancer, anti-metastasis and anti-recurrence

1) It was found from experimental tumor research in our laboratory as the following six points:

1. **A. Our laboratory removes the thymus (Thymus, TH) of mice (30), which can create cancer-bearing animal models.**
   B. Injection of immunosuppressive drugs can also help to establish cancer-bearing animal models.

The research conclusion proves:

The occurrence and development of cancer are obviously related to the host immune organ thymus and its function.

2. Is the immune system low first and then easy to get cancer, or is it the first to get cancer and then the immune system to start to decrease?

The results of the experiment are:

First, there is a low immunity, and then the occurrence and development of cancer occurs. If there is no decline in immune function, it is not easy to be successfully inoculated or vaccinated.

The results of this experiment suggest that improving and maintaining good immune function is one of the important measures to prevent cancer.

3. When we were studying the relationship between cancer metastasis and immunity, we established 60 animal models of liver metastasis and divided them into two groups A and B.

Group A uses immunosuppressive drugs, while group B does not.

The result:

The number of liver metastases in group A was significantly more than that in group B.

The results of this experiment suggest:

Metastasis is related to immune function. Low immune function or the application of immunosuppressive drugs may promote tumor metastasis.

4. When we were investigating the effects of tumors on the immune organs of the body, we found that as the cancer progresses, the thymus glands gradually shrink (600 cancer-bearing animal model mice).

The host's thymus glands show acute progressive atrophy after inoculation with cancer cells.

5. a. It was also found through experiments that in some experiments, If the mouse is not successfully inoculated or vaccinated, or the tumor is very small, the thymus gland does not shrink significantly.
   b. In order to understand the relationship between tumors and thymic atrophy, we removed solid tumors in a group of experimental mice when they grew to the size of a thumb, one month later, an autopsy revealed that the thymus had no further atrophy.

Therefore, we speculate that solid tumors may produce an unknown factor to suppress Thymus, which is looking for further experimental research.

6. The above experimental results prove:

The progression of the tumor can make the thymus progressively shrink. So, can we take some measures to prevent the atrophy of the host thymus?

Therefore, we further designed to find ways or drugs to prevent thymic atrophy in tumor-bearing mice through animal experiments. So we used the transplantation of immune organ cells to restore the function of the immune organ in experimental research.

During exploring the prevention of atrophy of the immune organ thymus during the tumor progression, finding the ways to restore the function of the thymus, and rebuilding the immune system, the transplantation of fetal liver, spleen, and thymus cells was carried out with mice, and the experimental study of the adoptive immune function were reconstructed.

The results showed that: S, T, and L cell transplantation (200 experimental mice), the recent complete tumor regression rate was 40%, the long-term complete tumor regression rate was 46.67%, and those with complete tumor regression achieved long-term survival.

2) ***The research on the effect of the new medication for anti-cancer metastasis which were searched and screened from Chinese medicine***

The results of the anti-tumor screening experiment on 200 kinds of traditional "anti-cancer Chinese medicine" tumor-bearing animals showed that:

a. *Among them, 48 species have inhibitory effects on cancer cells.*
   After optimized combination, the XZ-C $_{1-10}$ anti-cancer Chinese medicine preparation is formed by in vivo tumor suppression experiments in tumor-bearing animal models such as liver cancer, lung cancer and gastric cancer.

b. *XZ-C 1 can significantly inhibit cancer cells, but does not affect normal cells; XZ-C4 can promote thymic hyperplasia and increase immunity; XZ-C8 can protect the marrow to produce blood and protect the hematopoietic function of the bone marrow.*

c. *XZ-C immune regulation and control Chinese medicine can improve the quality of life of patients with advanced cancer, increase immunity, enhance the body's anti-cancer ability, enhance physical fitness, increase appetite, and significantly prolong survival.*

d. *We also used a mouse abdominal muscle transplantation tumor model (40 experimental mice) to observe the inhibitory effect of the Chinese herbal medicine Huangla Acetate Acetate Acetate Extract (TG) on the neovascularization of transplanted tumors in the abdominal muscles of mice and found out the traditional Chinese medicine TG that can inhibit tumor blood vessel formation.*

On the road of humans conquering cancer, research and development of effective anti-cancer, anti-cancer and anti-metastasis Chinese herbal medicines must be very promising.

All experimental research must pass clinical verification. In a large number of patients, observation for 3-5 years, or even clinical observation for 8-10 years, according to evidence-based medicine, with long-term follow-up and evaluable data, it is clear that there is indeed a good long-term effect.

All experimental research must pass clinical verification.

It must conduct observation on a large number of patients for 3-5 years, even clinical observation 8-10 years, according to evidence-based medicine, there are long-term follow-up and evaluable data, it verifies that it has ***sure long-term effective*** or confirms that the evidence is clear and indeed good Long-term curative effect.

*<u>**The goal of curative effect is:**</u>*
*<u>**good storage quality and long survival period.**</u>*

3

The introduction of these experiments in the experimental laboratory (with some pictures in details)

1) *Experimental study on non-tum or tumor-free technique during radical resection or operation*

Preventing postoperative cancer metastasis and recurrence must start from the operation, in other words, the prevention of Cancer Metastasis and Recurrence after operation must be made in Operation

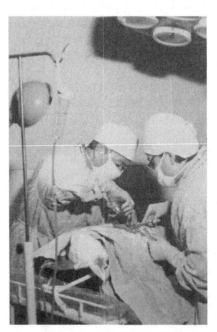

Professor Xu Ze (left)

This experiment is for research on intraoperative tumor-free technology:

This experiment is to study the intraoperative tumor-free technology to carry out the cancer-bearing animal model, and the experimental observation research during the operation. The Intraoperative observation of cancer cell shedding count and tumor cell detection and count in the vein blood of the tumor is done. Also observation of Staining and Tracking Experiment of Gastric Lymph Nodes is done. That is, *this experiment is to research the non-tumor technic in operation and make the experimental observation and research in operation through the cancer-bearing animal model. It was to observe the number of the exfoliative cancer cells, detect and number the cancer cells in the venous blood of tumor in operation. It was to perform experimental observation of the dyeing of the gastric lymph nodes by tracing.*

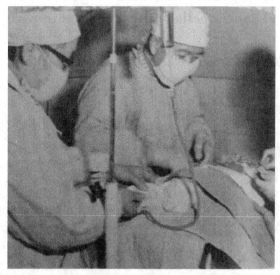

(Dr. Xu in the right side)

2) <u>**The Experimental Surgery Laboratory on Garden Hill is an animal laboratory in a two-story building.**</u>

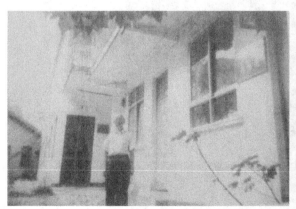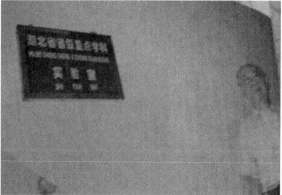

Dr. Xu Ze in the front of the research building

It was created by Professor Xu Ze in 1980, and established the actual scientific research exchange. It was undertook 15 scientific research projects including the Committee, the Ministry of Health, the Central Blood Office, the Chinese Academy of Medical Sciences, the Provincial Science and Technology Commission, and the Provincial Health Department. It was to train 10 postgraduates for Hubei University of Traditional Chinese Medicine, and to train two Ph.D. graduates for Tongji Medical College. It published 206 scientific research papers, and it obtained a number of scientific research achievements, two of which won the second prize of Hubei Science and Technology Achievement, and one Won the first prize of Hubei Provincial Department of Health.

3) **The series of observing ultrastructural organization or structure in the experimental model cancer cells with electron microscope**

Ultrastructure of H22 hepatocarcinoma cells in cancer-bearing mice

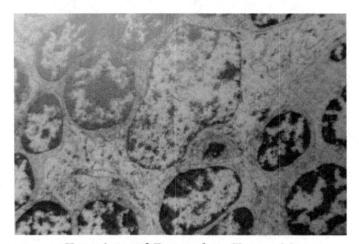

Experimental Research on Tumor A1

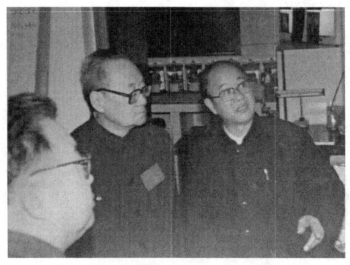

Academician Mao Shoubai (middle), vice president of the Chinese Academy of Preventive Medicine, and deputy leader of the United Nations Parasitology Group, came to inspect the experimental surgery laboratory.

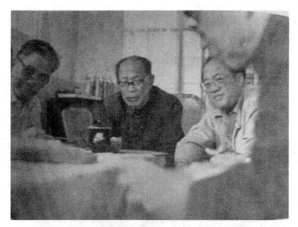

Academician Qiu Fazu (middle), the honorary president of Tongji Medical University, and the master of general surgery in my country, guides scientific research and design in the experimental surgery laboratory.

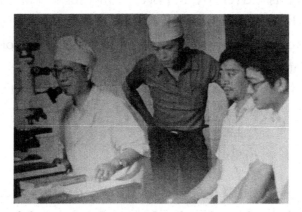

Professor Xu Ze (left 1), master's research soil (right 1), doctoral student (right 2)
Prof Xu Ze (Left I), doctor (Right 2)
Postgraduates (Right 1).

<u>*Tumor Experimental Research B1*</u>

Experimental Surgery Institute, anti-cancer metastasis and recurrence experiment

Experimetl on Anti-cancer Metastasis and Recurrence in Experimental Surgery Research Institute

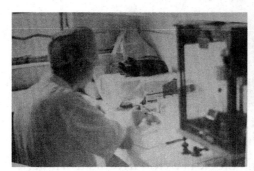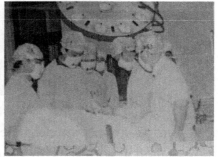

Tumor Experimental Research B2

Thymus atrophy in cancer-bearing mice

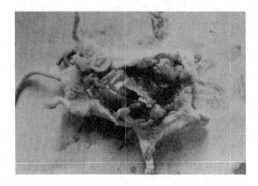

Experimental surgery is extremely important in the development of medicine. It is a key to open the forbidden area of medicine, or to open up the out-of- bounds area of the medical science. The preventive and curing ways of many diseases are applied to the clinic only when the stable achievements have been made through the experimental research on animals for many times, which promote the development of the medical science

Tumor Experimental Research B3

Animal Model for Experimental Research on Anti-cancer Metastasis and Recurrence

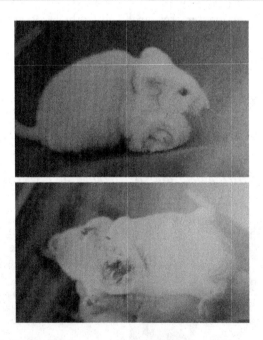

In a cancer-bearing animal model, one cancerous lump has fallen off or cancer-bearing animal model, with the cancerous block is exfoliative as a whole.

Tumor Experimental Research B4

Experimental oncology is the basic science of cancer prevention and treatment, which promotes the continuous and in-depth development of cancer research in my country. Without breakthroughs in basic research, it is difficult to improve clinical efficacy. Or the experimental Oncology is the fundamental science for prevention and treatment of tumor and promotes the further sustainable development of the research on cancer in China.Without the breakthrough of the fundamental research, it is difficult to improve the clinical curative effect.

T. S. L. Treatment of H22 liver cancer in cancer-bearing mice

Treatment of Cancer-bearing Mouse with H22 Liver Cancer with T.S.L.

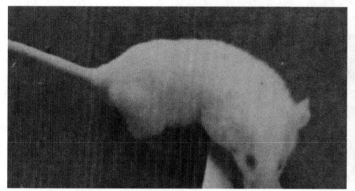 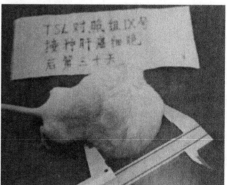

Left The treatment group   Right The control group

Tumor Experimental Research B5

ATCA treatment of S180 sarcoma tumor-bearing group, or treatment of tumor-bearing group with S180 Sarcoma with ATCA

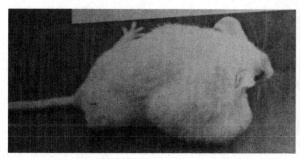 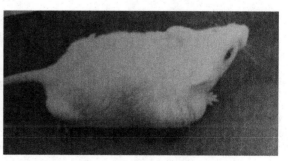

The group of control group   The group of treatment

The tumor experimental research B6

Observation of Inheritance of Cancer on Cancer-bearing Mouse through Disemboweling to take the fetus after conception as the following pictures:

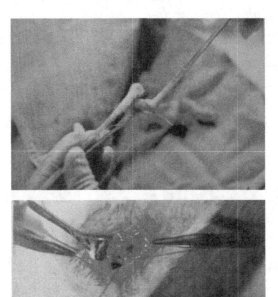

Tumor Experimental Research D1

Take the path of modernization of Chinese medicine, promote the integration of Chinese and Western medicine at the molecular level, and integrate with international medicine modernization

Immune regulation anti-cancer, anti-metastasis Chinese medicine series natural preparations

XZ-C Series Natural Medicine Preparation

- Self-developed XZ-C (XU ZE-Chiria) (Xu Ze-China) preparation
- Apply to clinical practice on the basis of 3 years of successful animal experiments.
- After 16 years of clinical verification by more than 12,000 clinical patients, the curative effect is remarkable.
- It is the result of independent invention, independent innovation and independent intellectual property rights.

Tumor Experimental Research D1

A. The Series Products of XZ-C Medicine

XZ-C immune regulation anti-cancer and anti-metastasis Chinese medicine series products

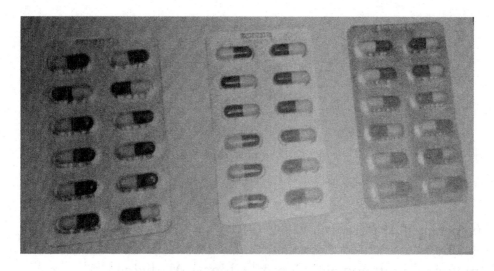

Tumor Experimental Research D2

B. The series Products of XZ-C Medicine

XZ-C immune regulation anti-cancer and anti-metastasis Chinese medicine series products

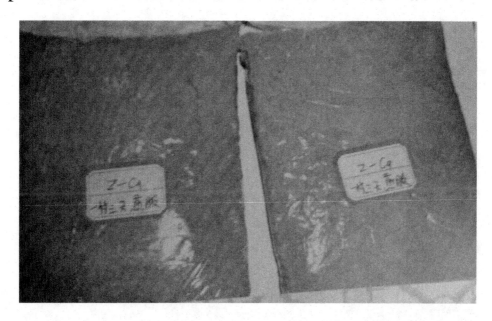

Tumor Experimental Research D3

C. The series Products of XZ-C Medicine

XZ-C immune regulation anti-cancer and anti-metastasis Chinese medicine series products

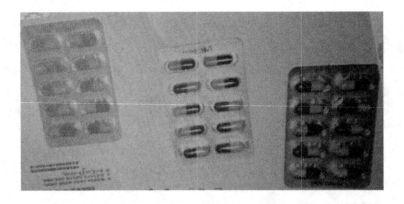

Tumor Experimental Research D4

XZ-C Immune Regulation and Control Chinese Medicine

The experimental study on Thymus protection and increase immune function as well as well as protecting Bone Marrow and Hematopoiesis(bone marrow protection) by XZ-C Medication as the following:

Treatment Group of XZ-C1 Medication and Control Group

[Control Group adopts CTX(cyclophosphamide)]
15 days after inoculation of liver cancer H22

XZ-C1 treatment group   The control group

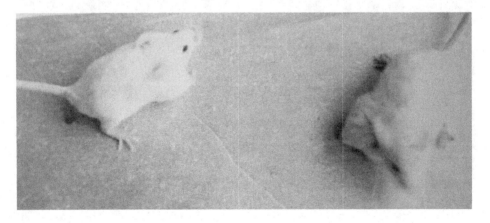

20 days after inoculation of liver cancer H22 as the following:

Tumor Thymus spleen kidney liver

The control group

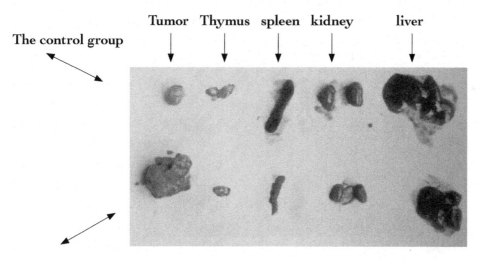

XZ-C1 treatment group

Experimental Research on Tumor D5

Treatment group and control group of XZ-C5 medication [the control group adopts CTX(cyclophosphamide)]

20 days after inoculation with liver cancer cells H22
XZ-C4 Treatment group   Control group

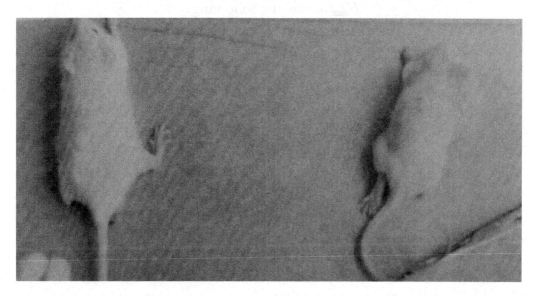

Treatment Group and control Group of XZ-C4 Medicine [Control Group adopts CTX(cyclophosphamide)]

20 days after inoculation of liver cancer H22

Control group

Tumor Thymus spleen kidney Liver

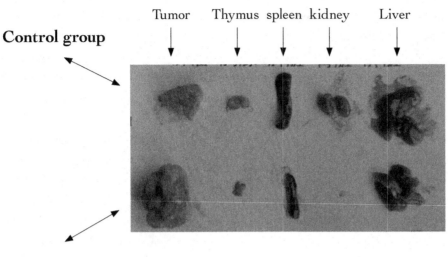

XZ-C4 treatment group

Experimental Research on Tumor D6

XZ-C5 treatment group and control group
The control group uses CTX (cyclophosphamide)

15 days after XZ-C inoculation with liver cancer

H22 are as the following:

XZ-C5 Treatment group   **The control group**

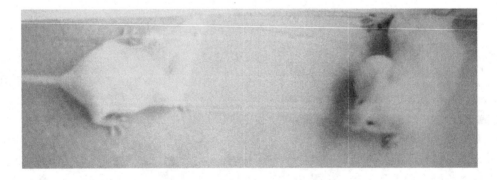

15 days after XZ-C inoculation with liver cancer
H22 are as the following:

Tumor Thymus spleen kidney liver

Control gruop

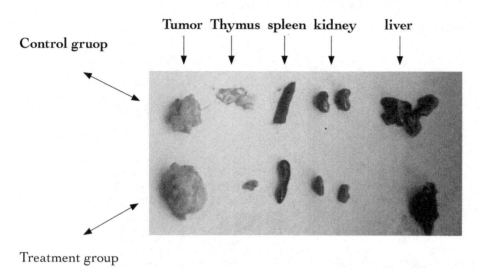

Treatment group

Experimental Research on Tumor E1

The exhibition board of scientific research results for "New Concepts and New Methods of Cancer Metastasis Treatment"

All are independent innovation and independent knowledge rights or intellectual

Being of independent Innovation and Independent Intellectual Property

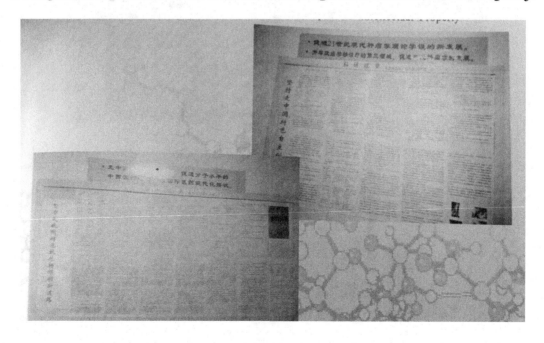

Experimental Research on Tumor E2

The Exhibition Board of Research Achievement for Anti-cancer, Anti-Metastasis and Anti-recurrence

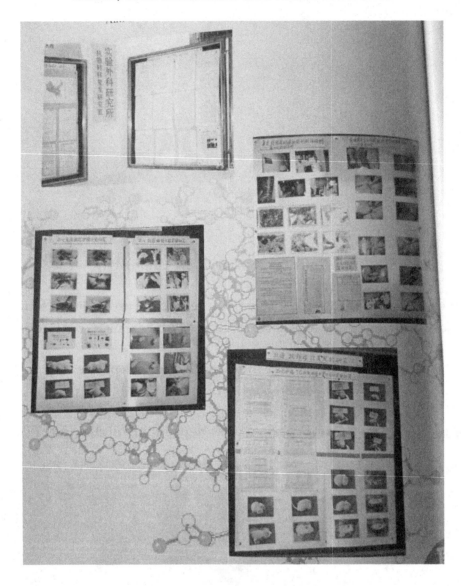

4

The research projects which were carried out as the following: (Research topics undertaken)

1) Experimental study and clinical observation of anti-metastasis of Chinese medicine Shenlu combined with advanced gastric cancer and liver cancer

------ Department of Traditional Chinese Medicine, Provincial Department of Health (Project leader: Xu Ze)

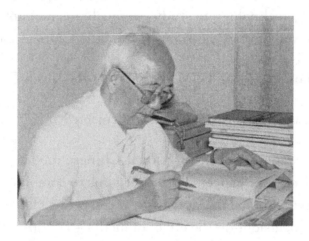

2) Clinical and experimental research on treatment of precancerous lesions of gastric cancer with traditional Chinese medicine

---------Special contract of National Science and Technology Commission, "Eighth Five-Year" National Science and Technology Research Plan
(Person in charge of the topic: Xu Ze)

3) Research on the mechanism of gastric cancer cell metastasis

----------National Natural Science Foundation of China
(Project owner: Xu Ze)

4) To further explore the experimental and clinical research of anti-cancer and cancer prevention Chinese herbal medicines on liver cancer, gastric cancer and pre-cancerous lesions of gastric cancer and anti-cancer metastasis with integrated traditional Chinese and western medicine

Key scientific and technological research projects during the "Eighth Five-Year Plan" period of the National Science and Technology Commission
(Project owner: Xu Ze)

5) Experimental research and clinical observation of allogeneic embryo thymus and/ or fetal spleen cell transplantation adoptive immunotherapy for advanced cancer

Hubei Provincial Party Committee, key scientific and technological research projects
(project leader: Xu Ze)

6) Experimental and clinical research on anti-cancer postoperative metastasis of Chinese medicine.

Use molecular biology technology to study the mechanism of anti-cancer metastasis of Chinese medicine and develop new anti-metastatic Chinese medicine

"Ninth Five-Year Plan" National TCM Technology Research Project

(Person in charge of the Hubei Collaboration Project: Xu Ze)

7) Research on the preparation of traditional Chinese medicine for interventional therapy of advanced liver cancer. This topic aims to combine traditional Chinese medicine with interventional therapy, anti-cancer, protect liver, promote immunity, and draw clear conclusions on the effect of media + traditional Chinese medicine in the treatment of liver cancer and attenuation of side effects

(Person in charge of the Hubei Association: Xu Ze)

5

The summary table for our research course

The research on one of the new concepts and new methods of anti-cancer metastasis therapy

---

In 1985, I sent letters and visits to more than 3,000 postoperative patients with chest and abdomen cancer.

The results found that: recurrence and metastasis are the key factors affecting the long-term efficacy of the operation.

↓

How to prevent and treat recurrence and metastasis requires basic clinical research

↓

So we established an animal laboratory

↓

Create cancer-bearing animal models

Our laboratory has the following new discoveries

↓

Experiment found 1: Removal of the thymus (Thymus) can create a cancer animal model.	Experimental finding 2: The use of immunosuppressive drugs to make immunity is conducive to the creation of cancer animal models.	Experiment found 3: As the cancer progresses, the thymus undergoes a contraction.	Experiment found 4: Cancer metastasis is related to immunity, and weak immune function may promote tumor metastasis.	Experiment found 5: In the inoculated mice, the thymus glands progressively atrophy; when not inoculated, the thymus glands do not shrink, and grow to the size of a fingertip, and the thymus glands no longer shrink.	Experiment found 6: Tumors can inhibit Thymus (TH) and cause atrophy of immune organs. Therefore, we believe that solid tumors may produce an unknown factor to inhibit TH, which is estimated to be called "cancer suppressor factor"

The above experimental results in our laboratory suggest:
Tumor progression causes the following:

1. It can make Thy mus progressively shrink.
2. It can make the body's immune function progressively decline.

How to prevent TH from shrinking?
How to promote immune surveillance?
Our laboratory has carried out the following research work:

How to keep Thymus from shrinking? How to keep immunity from exhaustion?	How to stop Thymus from shrinking? How to protect immune organs? How to avoid immune failure?
We adopt fetal liver, fetal thymus, and fetal spleen cell transplantation, adoptive immunization, and reconstruct its immune function.	We are looking for drugs to prevent thymus atrophy and increase immunity from Chinese medicine resources.
The results showed that the combined transplantation of S. T and L three groups of cells has a short-term complete tumor regression rate of 40%, and a long-term tumor regression rate of 46.67%. Those who have resolved will survive for a long time with good results.	So we conducted an experimental screening of 200 kinds of Chinese medicines, looking for Chinese medicines that protect the chest and promote immunity, protect the marrow of blood, and resist recurrence and transfer.
Experimental papers cannot be published	After 3 years of laboratory screening experiments: 1. In vitro tumor inhibition rate screening test tube experiment; 2. Screening experiment of tumor inhibition rate in cancer-bearing animal
It is shifted to using Chinese medicine as a resource, screening and searching natural medicines through animal experiments.	

6

The article I

**The experimental research of exploring the cause,
pathogenesis and pathophysiology of cancer and of searching
the effective measures for regulation and control**

As a result of follow-up, it was found that the questions or the problems or issues:

The recurrence and metastasis after surgery was the key to determine the long-term efficacy.

In another word, due to the findings of the follow-up, the problems which are found are:

The postoperative recurrence and metastasis are the key to determining the long-term effect of surgery

Thus, query the questions:

How to prevent and to treat the postoperative recurrence and metastasis?

How Clinical surgeons should pay attention to and study the prevention and treatment of postoperative recurrence and metastasis?

In other words, the question is raised that, **how the clinical surgeons should pay attention to and study the prevention and treatment measures for postoperative recurrence and metastasis?**

In 1985, the author petition more than 3,000 cases of all kinds of cancer patients whom the author had operated on for the general surgery and thoracic surgery.

The results of the follow-up found that vast majority of patients or most patients relapsed and metastasized within 2-3 years after surgery; some even died after recurrence and metastasis within a few months after surgery.

From this I thought that the operation was successful, but the long-term treatment was unsatisfactory or failed.

The patient underwent a major operation and only lived for 1-2 or 2-3 years.

Obviously this is not the request and purpose of the patient's treatment, nor is it what the doctor wants to see.

Usually we read the literature only pay attention to the 5-year survival rate and not the 5-year mortality rate.

For example, a group of gastric cancer has 20% of 5-year survival rate, and the 5-year mortality rate is 80%.

› Such a high 5-year postoperative mortality rate shocked the patients and their families.

Through the results of a large number of follow-ups, an important problem was discovered:

> *Postoperative recurrence and metastasis are key factors*
> *affecting the long-term efficacy of surgery.*

Therefore, an important question is also raised:
The research on methods and measures to prevent and treat postoperative recurrence and metastasis is the key to determining the long-term efficacy of surgery and the key to improving the survival of patients after surgery.

Through the results of a large number of follow-ups, an important issue was discovered:
Postoperative recurrence and metastasis are the key factors affecting the long-term efficacy of surgery.

Therefore, an important question is also raised:
Studying the methods and measures to prevent and cure postoperative recurrence and metastasis is the key to determining the long-term curative effect of the operation and the key to improving the patient's postoperative survival.

The current postoperative recurrence and metastasis rate is still quite high. Of course, it is related to many factors such as tumor stage, grade, differentiation and immune function of the body.

There are still many patients who see recurrence and metastasis after surgery in the outpatient department.

In one week, the author found 40 patients in the outpatient clinic, that is, 15 patients had relapse after surgery.

A rough analysis of these cases showed that they all relapsed within a few months after surgery.

It can be seen that the prevention and treatment of postoperative recurrence and metastasis must start from the operation.

Since cancer resection surgery is susceptible or prone to residues, tumor cells are prone to implanting and spreading, and once there are residues or spreading, recurrence and metastasis are extremely prone to occur, and the consequences are often unimaginable.

Therefore, the implementation of tumor surgery must follow the basic principles of tumor surgery.

The principle of tumor-free technology in oncology surgery must be as strict as the principle of aseptic technology performed by surgeons, or even more stringent.

There are two main purposes for implementing the principle of ***tumor-free technology***:

One is to prevent spreading, and the other is to prevent implanting.

The key to determining the long-term effect of surgery is recurrence and metastasis.

In the 20th century, surgeons have made brilliant achievements in cancer surgical resection.

In the 21st century the research task of surgeons should be to ***prevent postoperative recurrence and metastasis*** in order to improve the long-term efficacy of surgical treatment.

Without breakthroughs in basic research, it is difficult to improve clinical efficacy.

If the exact and effective measures for recurrence and metastasis after surgery are studied and resolved, the surgical treatment of solid tumors will surely achieve brilliant achievements.

Therefore, in 1985, our clinical surgery laboratory established an experimental surgery laboratory to carry out experimental tumor research.

First, it is to explore the manufacture of experimental tumor models, and begin to move from clinical to basic experimental research.

It is to explore the etiology, pathogenesis, and metastasis of cancer, and to explore prevention and treatment methods from multiple links of cancer metastasis.

In the past 7 years, the research projects have been clinical problems, aiming to explain some clinical problems or solve some clinical problems through experimental research.

Through 7 years of animal experimental research, we have explored basic problems one by one, step by step, and carried out and completed the following experimental research work.

1. The experimental research on making animal models of cancer

Why do people get cancer?
In what state will the body get cancer?
Why do some people get cancer and some not get cancer in the same environment and under the same conditions?
Is it the internal cause?
Is it an external cause?
Or internal and external causes?
It should create or make the animal models with cancer to explore all of these questions:

1) *The experimental research of carrying out tumors and making animal models bearing cancer*

At that time, the author was the director of clinical surgery and the director of experimental surgery research office of the Affiliated Hospital of Hubei College of Traditional Chinese Medicine.

It is convenient for clinical ward and animal laboratory subject work to be coordinated and coordinated simultaneously.

On the one hand, a sterile tumor specimen was removed from the clinical operating table, and it was transplanted into experimental animals within half an hour of warm ischemia.

It was done more than 100 times (400 animals) without success.

Afterwards, ***we removed some of the mice's thymus (THC)*** and transplanted these cancer cells again, which were successful to be transplanted (210 animals), and ***some were injected with cortisone to reduce the immunity of the mice***, and the transplantation of these cancer cells was successful.

5 days after the thymus is cut and transplanted, soya bean nodules can grow in 5-6 days, and it will grow to a large thumb tumor in 10-21 days.

Transplanted cancer can survive for 3-4 weeks, but cannot be passed down.

1. Through this research, it was found that:
   Removal of Thymus in the mice can create a cancer-bearing animal model, and injection of cortisone can help create a cancer-bearing animal model.

2. The research conclusion proves:
   The occurrence and development of cancer are related to the host's body immunity, and have a very obvious relationship with the immune organs and immune organ tissue functions.

3. The results of this study confirm:
   The immune organ thymus (Thymus, Th) and immune function have a very clear and positive relationship with the occurrence and development of cancer.

If the host Th is removed, it may be made into a cancer-bearing animal model. If it is not removed, it cannot be a cancer-bearing animal model.

Injection of immunosuppressive drugs to reduce host immunity will help create cancer-bearing animal models.

Without injection of anti-immunity drugs, cancer-bearing animal models cannot be created.

This result shows that immune organs and immunity are negatively correlated with cancer cell transplantation and implantation to grow into solid cancer.

Immunodeficiency or reduced immunity means transplantation can implant and grow tumors *that are not engulfed or swallowed by the host's immune cells.*

2) **Whether is it to have immune function decrease first, then to get cancer or to get cancer first and then get immune decrease?**

A total of 320 Kunming mice were divided into groups A, B, C, and D, n = 80 in each group.

Thymectomy (THC) and transplantation method were the same as before.

In group A, THC was removed first, and 10^6 cancer cells were inoculated 5 days later;

In group B, cortisone was injected first, and cancer cells were inoculated 7 days later:

Group C was inoculated with cancer cells first, and THC was removed 10 days later;

Group D was inoculated with tumor cells first, and cortisone was injected 10 days later.

The results are as the following:

Both groups A and B were successfully vaccinated and had developed small nodules;

In groups C and D, only 18 mice developed mung bean tumors after 14 days.

The results of this experiment suggest:

Tumors can only grow when the host's immune function is reduced or the immune organ thymus is defective.

If the host's immune function is good, it is not easy to grow tumors.

It can be concluded that:

First, the immune function is weakened and then cancer develops.

If there is no decline in immune function, it is not easy to be successfully vaccinated.

Tips from this research:

__Improving and maintaining good immune function and protecting well-functioning immune organs are important measures to prevent cancer.__

3) *__The modeling experiment of make the cancer metastasis model__*

1. Regarding cancer cell transplantation research, in 1985 we carried out dozens of human cancer cells transplanted into dethymic mice in the experimental surgery laboratory, and established solid cancer transplantation models.

2. Later, we made a cancer metastasis model to simulate lymphatic metastasis.
   We subcutaneously transplanted 106/ml 0.2ml, H22 CC. After 7-8 days, a broad bean-sized tumor grew on the inside of the foot pad, and the entire foot was swollen and encapsulated.

   16 days later, 8 mice found enlarged right inguinal lymph nodes and established **a lymphatic metastasis model.**

3. **After that, we simulated blood metastasis, injected H22 cell suspension 106/ ml 0.4ml into the vein for intravenous inoculation, and obtained more lung metastases, which caused tumor growth in the lung.**

4. **Later, an experimental animal model of liver metastasis was established.**
   80 Kunming mice were divided into two groups A and B, with 40 mice in each group.

Group A was injected with cortisone for 7 days, and all were anesthetized by intraperitoneal injection of 75 mg/kg of 1% barbitone, and then an incision of about 0.5 cm in length was made in the left middle abdomen to expose the spleen, and 10 ul of live H22 liver cancer ascites was taken and injected under the spleen capsule with local compression for 3-5 minutes to prevent cancer cells from spilling into the abdominal cavity and the spleen capsule.

After the animals were kept for 11 days, their necks were severed and their livers were taken for metastatic colony count.

The results are as the following:

There were liver cancer metastases in the liver of mice in groups A and B.

The number of metastases in the liver was different.

The number in group A was significantly more than that in group B, mostly more than 3 to 5, and the size was about 1mm.

In Group B the number is mostly 1 to 3.

The experimental results hint:

Metastasis is clearly related to immunity, and the immune function is low, or the application of immune suppression drugs can promote tumor metastasis.

2. **The experimental research of exploring the relationship between tumor and immune organs to seek the method of immune regulation and control**

While the laboratory is exploring the establishment of experimental cancer-bearing animal models, it has been found that removing the thymus or reducing immunity or making it immunodeficient can establish a cancer transplant animal model, so Th must be related to the growth of cancer inoculation, and the thymus is the central immune organ and the spleen is the largest immune organ in the periphery, so *__what is the relationship between the spleen and the tumor?__*

Therefore, we need to further design and study the relationship between immune organs and tumor occurrence and development, and conduct experimental research on the next subject.

1) **The experimental study on the effect of spleen on tumor growth**

In view of the fact that the spleen is a peripheral immune organ that has important immune functions and plays an important role in anti-tumor immunity, in order to explore the influence of the spleen, the largest peripheral immune organ, on tumor growth and its changes, the laboratory conducted the following experiments:

270 Kunming mice were divided into a spleen group and an without spleen group.

The spleenless group was further divided into the groups that one was inoculated with cancer cells and then cut the spleen, and another group was that the spleen was cut and then inoculated with cancer cells and then transplanted with spleen cells.

The results showed that the spleen had an inhibitory effect on tumor growth in the early stage of the tumor, with an inhibition rate of 25%.

In the late stage of the tumor, the progressive atrophy of the spleen would lose its inhibitory effect.

When the spleen cells was transplantation to the mice, *the spleen cell transplantation had an inhibitory effect on tumor growth, with an inhibition rate of 54%.*

The conclusions of this study are:

The effect of the spleen on tumor growth is biphasic. It has a certain inhibitory effect in the early stage and loses its inhibitory effect in the late stage.

The spleen cell transplantation can enhance the effect of inhibiting tumor growth.

2) *The experimental study on the effect of tumors on the body's immune organs of thymus and spleen*

In the previous experimental research, we have discussed the effects of the central immune organ, the thymus, and the spleen of the peripheral immune organs on cancer cell transplantation and tumor growth. The findings and conclusions of the experimental results are as described above.

So, in turn, think about it further, what effect will the tumor have on the immune organs thymus and spleen?

It is further designed and carried out the following experimental research:

Randomly divide 40 Kunming mice into 4 groups.

Blood was collected to measure the lymphocyte transformation rate before inoculation of cancer cells and on the 3rd, 7th and 14th days after inoculation of cancer cells, and sacrificed to observe the thymus, spleen and weigh them, and make cancer tissue sections or slides.

It turns out:

1. *The spleen:*

> In the early stage of tumor growth, the spleen is congested and enlarged, and cell proliferation is active.

> In the late stage of the tumor, the spleen shows progressive atrophy and cell proliferation is blocked.

2. *The Thymus:*

> After the thymus was inoculated with cancer cells, it immediately showed acute progressive atrophy, cell proliferation was blocked, the volume was significantly reduced, and the weight was significantly reduced, indicating that the cellular immune function was suppressed.

The results of this experiment suggest:

> Tumors can significantly inhibit the thymus, not only inhibiting the function of the thymus, but also causing atrophy of immune organs.

3. The experimental study of exploring the methods of curbing thymic atrophy during tumor progression and finding methods for immune reconstruction

A.

When we made the cancer-bearing animal model above, we found that only THC can be successfully made, and repeated the same experiment in 3 batches.

The results clearly prove:

Thymus has a positive relationship with tumor occurrence.

B.

In the above experimental studies on the relationship between tumors and immune organs, the results clearly prove:

The progression of the tumor can quickly cause Thyrnus to shrink progressively, indicating that the tumor significantly inhibits the thymus, *not only inhibiting its function, but also causing atrophy of immune organs*.

If this is the case, can we use some methods to prevent the host's thymus from shrinking, restore the function of the thymus, and rebuild the immune system?

Therefore, we further designed and wanted to use the immune organ cell transplantation to restore the immune organ and rebuild its organ function. We carried out an experimental study of adoptive immunity to reconstruct its immune function by transplantation of fetal liver, spleen and thymocytes.

A closed group of 200 Kunming mice was used to create a subcutaneous solid carcinoma model of Hey's ascites carcinoma, divided into 6 experimental groups and 2 control groups, and transplanted fetal spleen cells, fetal thymocytes, and fetal liver cells respectively.

The tumor growth, regression, survival time, cellular immune indexes and various histopathological examinations were systematically observed in each group of mice, and the efficacy of each group was compared.

The results showed that the three groups of cell transplantation, the short-term complete tumor regression rate was 40%, the long-term complete tumor regression rate was 46.67%, and those with complete tumor regression achieved long-term survival.

The partial remission rate is 26.67% in the short term and 13.33% in the long term.

The survival period of some people who have regressed was extended by an average of more than one month, the immune indicators were significantly improved, and the immune organs were enlarged.

Tissue slides or sections of immune organs showed active cell proliferation.

The results of this experiment show that:

Compared with partial reconstruction, systemic adoptive immune reconstruction can better exert its anti-elbow tumor immune function and improve curative effect through the overall synergy of the system.

4. look for drugs that inhibit tumor neovascularization from natural drugs

In 1986, when cancer cells were cultured in our laboratory, they could only promote the growth of cancer cells, but could not form solid tumor masses.

During the experiment, we accidentally discovered that if 1 to 2 drops of chicken soup were added to the culture of test-tube cancer cells, it would promote the rapid growth of cancer cells into clusters, and if 1-2 drops of aminophylline were added, they would spread out quickly.

Since then we have been admonishing cancer patients not to eat chicken.

Currently, it is known that cancer cell metastasis has several steps:

First, the cancer cells fall off, then invade the blood vessels and enter the bloodstream, through the bloodstream to reach the microcirculation and then invade the capillaries, reach the metastatic organs, implantation. At the beginning there is an avascular stage and the tumor exists as the tumor nodule, which will not grow up, and then the new blood vessels are formed quickly, and the tumor grows rapidly.

In this metastasis process, if one of the links can be blocked, then tumor metastasis can be prevented. We consider the formation of new tumor microvessels, which is one of the key links in whether metastatic cancer cells can implant and grow into cancer nodules.

Therefore, it is an experimental study designed to find anti-tumor angiogenesis drugs from natural drugs.

1) ***The experimental study on observation of neovascularization of tumors transplanted into abdominal muscles in mice***

Twenty Kunming mice were inoculated with EAC cell fluid into the abdominal muscles to create an animal model of tumor neovascularization in abdominal muscle transplantation.

The Olympus microcirculation photomicrography system was used to observe the formation of new microvessels and count the flow rate and flow of microvessels.

It turns out:

On the first day after inoculation there was no new blood vessels.

On the second day, the new blood vessels from the original host's microvessels were seen to enter the tumor.

On the 3-4 days, the density of new blood vessels outside the tumor increased.

2) ***The experimental study on the effect of different doses of Huang Lateng ethyl acetate extract (TG) on the immune function of mice***

Kunming rats were randomly divided into TG1 group, TG2 group, TG3 group, TG4 group and other different dose experimental groups for 40 days.

Different doses of TG were intragastrically administered for 12 days.

On the 13th day, the rats in each group were sacrificed, and the thymus and spleen were weighed.

It turns out:

Different doses of TG have different effects on the immune organs of young mice.

A small dose of 20 mg/kg can increase the weight of the thymus, and a large dose of 30 mg/kg can atrophy the thymus.

3) ***The experimental study of the inhibitory effect of Huang Lateng ethyl acetate brewing extract ((TG) on the neovascularization of abdominal muscle transplantation tumor in mice***

To observation of neovascularization of abdominal muscle tumor by inoculating EAC with 40 Kunming mice in the abdominal muscles:

1. Place the mouse on the self-made observation platform, then put the mouse observation platform on the microscope stage in the incubator, and observe the shape and number of new microvessels in and around the tumor with the HH-1 type microcirculation detection system.
2. And take a photomicrograph to measure the density of new microvessels entering and exiting the tumor and the average diameter and flow velocity of the arteries and veins of the tumor.

The results showed that:

In the early stage of tumor, TG (20mg/kg) significantly inhibited tumor angiogenesis.

From the results of this group of experiments, TG can significantly inhibit the growth of new microvessels in and around the tumor, and reduce the density of new microvessels entering and leaving the tumor.

At present, scholars at home and abroad are paying attention to trying to inhibit tumor neovascularization to control tumor growth and metastasis formation.

Folkman in the United States reported in May 1998 that his laboratory had developed two drugs that inhibit tumor neovascularization: ***angiostatin and endostatin***.

In the tumor-bearing animal experiment, the tumors transplanted into the test mice from the human body were significantly reduced.

He used this anti-angiogenesis inhibitor to prevent the growth of blood vessels, shrink the capillaries and cut off the nutritional supply of the tumors so as to achieve the purpose of treating cancer.

They reported plans to conduct very limited experiments on humans in 1999.

Our laboratory completed the above-mentioned experimental study of TG in July 1997 because TG is a traditional Chinese medicine.

This Chinese medicine has been used in Chinese medicine books for hundreds of years, and it has been used in clinical practice for a long time. However, it has never been used in treatment to inhibit the growth of new biological blood vessels in tumors.

So since September 1998, we have tried to use it in clinical outpatients as one of the comprehensive anti-cancer and anti-metastasis comprehensive treatments. Since December 1999, it has been used in more than 80 patients with stage II and III cancers.

The preliminary observation conclusions on the curative effect of the control, recurrence, and metastasis are good, **and it is currently under clinical verification and observation.**

7

The article Two

The experimental observation on the effect of tumor on immune organs thymus and spleen

It is generally believed that *the body's immune function affects* the occurrence, development and prognosis of tumors.

At the same time, *tumors also inhibit the immune status of the body.*

The two are causal to each other and intricate.

During our animal experiment on the effect of spleen on tumor growth, we observed many changes in the **thymus and spleen of** the immune organs of tumor-bearing mice.

It seems that there is a certain pattern of performance during this period.

In order to further explore the relationship between the tumor and the spleen and thymus and their regularity, the following experiment was designed to dynamically observe the changes in *the thymus, spleen, and lymphocyte transformation rates of tumor-bearing mice in different periods and explore the regularity between them.*

1. Materials and methods

1) The laboratory animals and grouping

Forty Kunming mice were randomly divided into 4 groups, aged 40-50 days, and weighing 15-18g. Male and female are irrelevant.

Group I:

The healthy control group, healthy mice not inoculated with cancer cells. Thymus, spleen and peripheral blood were taken for experimental observation after execution.

Group II:

Inoculated with 0.1×10^7 Ehrlich ascites carcinoma through the abdominal cavity, and sacrificed for observation 3 days later.

Group III:

inoculated with cancer cells (same as above), and sacrificed on the 7th day for observation.

Group IV:

on the 14th day of inoculation with cancer cells, they were sacrificed for observation.

Take the autopsy results of 100 tumor-bearing mice after spontaneous terminal death in the first part of the experiment (the experimental study of the effect of the spleen on tumor growth) as the result of the changes **in the thymus and spleen of advanced cancer.**

The average diameter of **the thymus** in late-stage tumor-bearing mice is about 1.2±0.3 mm, the average weight is about 20±5 mg, and the texture is hard.

The **spleen** is extremely atrophic, with an average weight of about 60±12 mg, hard texture, grayish-white color, significantly reduced germinal centers, and fibrosis.

2) *The Experimental method*

Mice in each group were put to death by eyeballs and bloodletting at the planned time. In other words, the mice in each group were put to death by eyeballing and bleeding at the scheduled time.

1ml of whole blood (anticoagulated with heparin) was collected from each mouse for lymphocyte transformation test.

Then the mice were immediately dissected to observe the tumor infiltration range and ascites volume and the involvement of various organs.

The anatomy of the *thymus, spleen, and lymph nodes* was observed macroscopically.

The thymus and spleen were taken out completely, and the volume was measured with a vernier caliper.

Then, the weight was weighed with an analytical balance and sent for medical examination.

3) **The determination of the conversion rate of peripheral blood lymphocytes in each group of mice**

The micro-volume whole blood morphology method was used for determination.

Pick the eyeball and take whole blood, heparin anticoagulation.

4) **Tumor model preparation**

It is the same as the first part of the experiment.

2. The experimental results

1. The weight of the thymus of mice at different periods after inoculation with cancer cells is shown in Table 1.

It is to perform variance analysis on Table 1, see Table 2.

The results in Tables 1 and 2 are represented by curves, and the thymus weight change curve is drawn (Figure 1).

The weight of the thymus on the 25th and 30th day in the figure is from the results of the first part of the experiment.

Table 1

The comparison of the weight of thymus in each group of experimental mice

Unit: mg

Group	Group I normal group	Day 3 after group II inoculation	Day 7 after Group III inoculation	Day 14 after vaccination in group IV	
	72.8	78. 2	90.0	40. 0	
	50.0	83. 4	66.0	32.2	
	56.4	89	85. 4	39. 8	

96.4	68	106. 5	23. 5	
77. 4	74. 8	51.7	38.0	
100.7	95. 4	77. 8	36.0	
87.5	115. 0	73.0	46.0	
76.8	56. 4	60.0	20.0	
112.7	43.0	49.4	55	
51.0			20	
$\sum X$ 781. 07	703.2	736.3	350. 5	$\sum X$ **2571. 7**
Ni 10	**9**	**10**	**10**	**N 39**
$\bar{x}$ 78. 17	78. 13	73. 63	35. 05	$\sum \bar{x}$**133.59**
$\sum iX$ 66261. 79	58566. 66	57033. 75	18467. 25	$\sum X^2$**191324.75**

Table 2

Analysis of variance for Tables 1

Source of variation	SS	V	MS	F	P
Between groups	12967. 10	3	4322. 36	12. 85	<0.01
Within group	11777.12	35	336.48		
Total	**24744. 22**	**38**			

As can be seen from Table 1, Figure2, and Figure 1, Thymus in tumor-bearing mice showed regular changes:

Within 7 days after the inoculation, there was no obvious change in the thymus visual appearance, but the weight had begun to decrease.

After 7 days, it showed acute progressive atrophy, and the diameter of each leaf of the thymus decreased from the normal 5-8 mm to about 1 mm in the late stage.

The weight was reduced from 76.1 mg to 20 mg, and the texture became hard. As a result, the function is also reduced or even lost. It shows that the body's cellular immune function is increasingly manipulated and suppressed with the progress of the tumor, the immune function is low, and the tumor grows faster and faster.

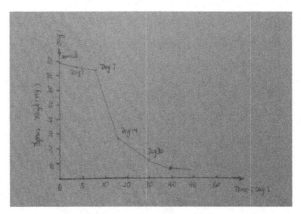

Figure 1. Thymus weight change curve

2. Changes in spleen weight of each group of tumor-bearing mice in different periods See table 3, 4.

Table 3

The spleen weight of each group of tumor-bearing mice at different stages

Unit: mg

Group	Group I normal group	Group II day 3 after inoculation	Group III day 7 after inoculation		Group IV day 14 after inoculation
	98.4	103.0	152.8		120.7
	86. 0	110. 3	175.8		96.9
	139.0	153. 2	154. 5		103.0
	126. 0	96. 7	154, 0		102.0
Xij	194.4 4	206. 0	290. 4		91.0
	130	137. 0	156. 0		122.3
	107. 4	174. 0	184. 0		88.6
	82. 8	143. 0	232. 0		109.0
	86. 0	160	86. 3		102.4
	82.0				119.0
X	1258.4	1209. 0	1720.09	1021 X	5210. 2
Ni	10	9	10	10 N	39
$\bar{x}$	125.24	134. 43	1720. 9	102. 1 $\bar{x}$	133. 59
$\sum iX^2$	169020. 88	175088.97	322834, 65	106.41 $\sum X^2$	773. 385

Table 4 The analyzes the variance of Table 3

Source of variation	SS	V	MS	F	P
Between groups	25345. 12	3	8448	5. 68	<0.01
Within group	11777.12	35	336.48		
Total	77 328. 12	38			

As mentioned above, the spleen influences tumor growth in 100 mice of the experimental group. The average weight of the spleen is 60 ± 12 mg. The weight change of the spleen is now described as a curve (Figure 2).

From Table 3 and Table 4. Figure 2, it can be seen that the spleen of the tumor-bearing mice gradually increased in volume and weight in the early stage, while progressively atrophy in the later stage. This indicates that during a dry period of tumors, due to tumor stimulation, the cells proliferate actively, the immune response effect is strengthened, the tumor suppressing effect is also strengthened, and it plays a role in inhibiting tumor growth. In the late stage, due to a large increase in the number of tumors, a large number of suppressor cells and immunosuppressive factors are produced, which inhibits the proliferation of spleen immune cells and the consumption of effector cells, and atrophy, fibrous tissue hyperplasia, tumor suppression effect weakens or disappears, and even promotes tumor growth.

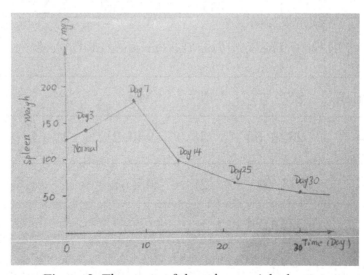

Figure 2. The curve of the spleen weigh changes

3. The comparison of the results of peripheral blood lymphocyte transformation test in tumor-bearing mice at different times. See Table 5 and Table 6 as the followings:

Table 5

The comparison of lymphocyte rate in different groups of lymphocyte transformation test at different times

Group I Normal group (%)		Group II Day 3 after inoculation in (%)	Group III Day 7 (%)	Group IV Day 14 (%)		
45		53	43	31		
40		62	32	28		
51		48	26	19		
42		43	45	21		
60		52	30	22		
39		51	32	23		
		50				
$\sum X$	277	1209. 0	1720.09	1021	X	5210. 2
Ni	6	17	6	6	N	25
$\bar{x}$	46.17	51.29	24		$\sum \bar{x}$	39.52
$\sum \bar{x}$	13111	18611	7498	3560	$\sum X^2$	42780

Table 6 The analyzes the variance of Table 5

Source of variation	SS	V	MS	F	P
Between groups	2820. 54	3	940. 21	21. 614	<0.01
Within groups	913. 59	21	43. 51		
Total	3734. 24				

The results of Tables 5 and 6 are represented by curves, and the lymphocyte transformation rate curves of tumor-bearing mice at different times are depicted. See Figure 3.

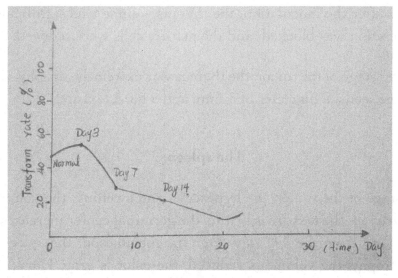

Figure 3. The curve of lymphocyte transformation rate

As can be seen from Table 5 and Figure 3, the change of lymphocyte transformation rate of tumor-bearing mice also showed a certain pattern, followed by an acute and progressive decline, and by the 14th day (late stage) after inoculation, the transformation rate fell to It is about 50% of normal, and it will continue to decline in the future, indicating that the tumor's cellular immune effect on the body has an inhibitory effect throughout the course of the disease, and as the disease progresses, the stronger the inhibitory effect, the more the immune function is damaged.

Combining table 5,6, and Figure 3, it can be seen that the volume-weight change curve of the thymus is very similar to the curve of lymphocyte transformation rate. Show synchronization. There is a difference between the spleen volume and weight change curve and the two. It increased once in the early stage and then decreased later. It shows that in the middle and late stages of the tumor, both the body's humoral and cellular immune functions are damaged and suppressed.

4. Pathological changes of thymus and spleen

The thymus:

The thymus showed progressive atrophy throughout the course of the disease.

On the 3rd day after the cancer cells were inoculated, the thymus was slightly shrunken and pale in color.

On the 7th day after the inoculation, the thymus volume was significantly atrophy, the cell proliferation was blocked, and the mature cells were reduced.

At the advanced stage of the tumor, the thymus was extremely atrophy, with a volume of about sesame seeds, a diameter of 1 mm, and a hard texture.

The spleen:

In the early stage of the tumor, the hyperemia and swelling, the volume increases, the color is dark red, the texture is brittle, the germinal center increases, the mature cells are few, and from the 14th day after the inoculation, the spleen also shows progressive atrophy, the volume is reduced, the color is gray, Hard, the germinal center is reduced, cell proliferation is blocked, mature cells are few, and fibrous hyperplasia occurs until fibrosis.

3. Discussion

1. *Regarding the impact or effect of tumors on the structure and function of the spleen*

The results of this experiment show that tumors affect the body's immune function status, and the spleen of tumor-bearing mice undergoes regular changes.

In the early stage, the spleen proliferates and enlarges, cell proliferation is active, germinal centers increase, and mature cells increase, which can inhibit tumor growth or play a role in inhibiting tumor growth.

In the late stage, the spleen shows progressive atrophy, cell proliferation is restricted, germinal centers are reduced, and fibrous tissue proliferates and fibrosis, the quality becomes hard, and the anti-tumor immunity is lost.

The mechanism of this change in the spleen is still unclear and needs to be further explored.

It may be speculated as follows:

On the one hand, tumor cells stimulate the host's immune system through tumor-specific antigens to stimulate immune effects to kill tumor cells, thereby clearing them, and protecting the body.

On the other hand, tumor cells can induce the inhibition of the production of immune cells (mainly T suppressor cells and macrophages) and the production of the suppressor factors.

In addition, tumor cells themselves secrete many immunosuppressive factors, thereby suppressing the body's immune and anti-cancer effects, and escape the effect of immune killing and guardianship and survive and develop.

The spleen is the body's largest peripheral lymphatic organ, which can produce immune lymphocytes and antibodies, and can produce humoral molecules with anti-tumor effects-Tuft is in.

When cancer cells invade the body in the early stage, the spleen is stimulated to respond, and the cells proliferate and function vigorously, producing more immune effector cells and lymphokines to inhibit tumor growth.

In the late stage, due to the progress of cancer, a large number of immunosuppressive factors are produced, which leads to atrophy of the spleen, restricted or damaged functions, and thus loses the positive effect of anti-tumor immunity.

2. About the impact of tumor on the thymus

The experimental results show that:

After the cancer cells were inoculated, the thymus was immediately suppressed, and the whole process was atrophy, so the thymus immediately lost the anti-tumor immune effect.

It was observed in the experiment that the thymus had some morphological changes soon after the cancer cells were inoculated, and the entire course of the disease was progressively atrophied.

To the late stage of the tumor, the weight of the thymus was reduced from 78.13 ± 13.2 mg to 20 + 5 mg, and the volume was reduced from 5-8 to 1 mm in diameter.

The cell proliferation was significantly hindered.

Due to the progressive atrophy of the thymus, the proliferation of paper cells is blocked, the mature cells are reduced or exhausted, the index decreases, the metabolism is weakened, and the cell viability is reduced.

In addition, the secretion of thymus hormones is also reduced, and the body's cellular immune function must be damaged. The defense ability of the mouse is low, and the transplanted cancer cells grow and reproduce in large numbers.

Similar reports have been made by Zhang Tongwen and others that they found that the tumor-bearing mice had atrophy of the thymus, which was accompanied by the proliferation of bone marrow cells and the decline of nucleated cell viability. They believed that there was a close relationship between the two. It can be seen that the inhibition or damage of the tumor on the host's immune function is multi-faceted, affecting the entire immune system of the body.

The group's lymphatic transfection test showed that after inoculation of cancer cells, the lymphatic transfusion rate decreased progressively, and decreased to more than 50% in the late stage, which also showed that the cellular immune effect was suppressed. As for why the thymus of tumor-bearing mice is suppressed and atrophy, further experimental research and observation are needed.

In order to achieve immune function, vertebrates have evolved to have a special lymphatic network system distributed throughout the body,

The entire immune system is composed of central lymphoid organs and peripheral lymphoid organs.

__The thymus is an important central lymphoid organ, which promotes the differentiation and maturation of T cells to play a role in cellular immunity and complement B cells to produce antibodies. The thymus also produces a variety of thymic hormones to promote the differentiation and maturation of immune lymphatic stem cells. Although the thymus is a lymphoid organ, due to the presence of the blood thymus barrier, the thymus does not directly contact with antigenic substances and exerts an effect. Therefore, it is not stimulated by tumor-specific antigens and hyperplasia__. However, the *__tumor produces secretory immunosuppressive factors__* that can act on the thymus, causing it to shrink progressively and impair its function.

For immunotherapy of malignant tumors, many doctors are devoted to the development of this field with great interest.

As early as 1968, Krant et al reported that the cellular immune function of patients **with lung cancer** was suppressed, and the patients had a delayed allergic reaction to dinitrochlorobenzene (DNCB) and pure tuberculin (PPD). And it was found **that**

the body's immune system damage is getting more and more serious as the tumor progresses.

Over the past 20 years, the relationship between the body's immune status and the occurrence, development, and prognosis of tumors has increasingly attracted the attention of oncologists.

Since the 1980s, due to the rapid development of immunology and biotechnology, it has provided opportunities for immunotherapy for cancer patients.

The theory of biological response regulation has been proposed, and a fourth treatment program other than surgery, radiotherapy, and chemotherapy has been established.

That is tumor biological therapy (BRM). The use of biomodulators to treat tumors may hopefully lead to the development of new immunotherapies that are effective for tumors.

In short, **the host and the tumor are a pair of contradictions**, and have always existed throughout the entire process of tumor development.

When the body's immune system is functional, the body can respond to tumors through its cellular and humoral immune responses to limit and eliminate the tumor.

On the other hand, a growing tumor has many effects on the body's immune system, suppresses the body's immune function, and promotes the development of the tumor.

8

The article Three

The effect of spleen on tumor growth

The experimental study of the effect of spleen on tumor growth

In recent years, the role of the spleen in anti-tumor immunity has received increasing attention. Its anti-cancer effect is very complicated. There are still many differences and doubts.

In order to further explore the effect of the spleen on tumor growth and understand the relationship between the spleen and tumor immunity, we used experimental surgical methods to prepare Ehrlich ascites carcinoma models.

The spleen was removed before and after inoculation with cancer cells in the aspleen group and compared with the spleen group, the following experiment was performed to observe the effect of splenectomy on the tumor immune status.

1. Material method

1) The grouping of experimental animals

The Kunming species of white mice, male and female, are between 50 and 60 years old and weigh 15-20g, for a total of 300 mice.

According to the spleen and the spleen cut, the spleen cut and the inoculation of cancer cells are divided into 5 groups.

These mice are divided into 5 groups according to the mice with spleen and with spleen which is cut off, the spleen which is cut off in the difference time for doing the cancer cell inoculation, and according to the content of the inoculated cells (1×10^4ml or 1×10^7ml) and the inoculation site (abdominal cavity or subcutaneous), each group is divided into A and B subgroup.

The specific grouping is as follows:

Group I: the control group with spleen

It is to simulate spleen excision first, and inoculate 0.1ml of Ehrlich ascites cancer cells intraperitoneally or subcutaneously after 7 days, containing 1×10^4 or 1×10^7 cancer cells (Table 1)

Table 1

The control group with the simulated spleen cutting (group I)

Group I	Number of inoculated cancer cells	Inoculation site	mice (number)
I-A1	0.1x104	right armpit subcutaneous	15
I-A2	0.lx104	abdominal cavity	15
I-B1	0.1X107	right armpit subcutaneous	15
I-B2	0.1x10	abdominal cavity	15

Group II:
The group that the spleen was cut first and then inoculated with cancer cells.

The spleen was excised first and then subcutaneously or spleen cavity was inoculated Ehriich ascites cancer cells 0.1ml, containing 1×104 or 1×107 cancer cells (Table 2).

Group III:
It is also a spleen-free group.

The cancer cells are inoculated with cancer cells first and then cut the spleen 7 days later. All were inoculated subcutaneously in the right armpit, with a content of 1×104ml or 1×107ml (Table 3).

Table 2
The group that the spleen is cut first and then inoculated

Group II	Number of cancer cells inoculated	Inoculation site	mice (number)
II-A1	0.1x104	Right subaxillary skin	15
II-A2	0.1x104	abdominal cavity	15
II-B2	0.1X104	Right subaxillary skin	15
II-B2	0.1x104	abdominal cavity	15

Table 3
The group that the spleen is resected after inoculation of cancer cells

Group II	Number of cancer cells inoculated (number)	Inoculation site	mice (number)
III-A	0.1x104	Right subaxillary skin	15
III-B	0.1x10	Right subaxillary skin	15

Group IV:

To cut the spleen first, then inoculate cancer cells and then transplant spleen cells or spleen tissue clear fluid group:

The spleen was removed first.

Seven days later, cancer cells were inoculated, and one day later, live spleen cell suspension or spleen tissue supernatant was injected intraperitoneally (Table 4).

Table 4

The group that is cut the spleen first and then transplant
the spleen cell suspension or spleen supernatant

Group II	Number of cancer cells inoculated	Inoculation site	Processing factors	Mouse (number)
IV-A1	0.1 X104	right armpit	Injection of spleen supernatant	15
IV-A2	0.1 X104	Abdominal cavity	Injection of spleen supernatant	15
IV-B	10.1 X107	right armpit	Transplantation of splenocytes from newborn mice	15
IV-B2	0.1 X107	Abdominal cavity	Transplantation of splenocytes from newborn mice	15

Group V:

The compound group for strengthening the spleen and invigorating qi (Table 5).

Table 5

The compound group for strengthening the spleen and invigorating
qi by taking traditional Chinese medicine (without spleen cut)

Group V	Number of cancer cells inoculated	Inoculation site	Processing factors	Mice (number)
V-A	10X0.1	Right under the armpit	Take Chinese medicine for 10 days first, and continue taking the medicine for 3 weeks after vaccination	15
V-B	10X0.1	Right under the armpit	Take medicine for 3 weeks after vaccination	15

Table 6

The summary table of the experimental Animal Groups

Method of inoculation / Group	Cancer cell concentration 1X104/ml		Cancer cell concentration 1X107/ml	
	Percutaneous	Abdominal	Percutaneou	Abdominal
Group I (simulated spleen cut)	IA1 (15	I A2 (15)	I B1 (15)	IB2 (15)
Group II (first cut the spleen and then inoculate)	IIA1(15)	II A2(15)	IIB1(15)	IIB(15)
Group III (first vaccination and then spleen cut)	IIIA (30)		IIIB (30)	
Group IV (first cut the spleen and then inoculated+ spleen cell)	IVA1(15)	IV A2(15)	IVB1(15)	IVB2(15)
Group V (for Chinese medicine)	VA (15)		VB (15)	

2. Apparatus and materials

1) Animal sterile operating room and a set of sterile surgical instruments

2) Hank's solution, improved Hank's solution. Calf serum, PRH, tri-distilled water, normal saline for injection, ketamine, phenobarbital sodium, heparin sodium, placepan blue stain, Jimusari's stain, sodium bicarbonate hydrochloride, L-glutamine, Allergenic and non-allergenic zymosan.

3) 400prm centrifuge. Glass homogenizer, vibrator. Filter metal mesh (No. 1000), funnel, incubator, oven, low temperature water tank, microscope, relatively sterile workbench. (4) Animal feed, refined pellet feed.

Drinking water: tap water.

Feeding cage: plastic squirrel cage.

3. Tumor inoculation and model preparation

The Ehrfich ascites cancer cancer strain was introduced from the cell room of Wuhan Institute of Biology.

The ascites containing cancer cells were extracted from the abdominal cavity of the mice with Ehrlich ascites cancer and ascites tumor animals, and they were washed and centrifuged 3 times with modified Han k's solution at a centrifugal speed of 800 Prm for 5 minutes.

The supernatant was discarded, and Hank's solution was used to prepare the precipitated cancer cells into a cancer cell suspension containing 1×104ml or 1×107ml of cancer cells, respectively.

The viable cell rate was confirmed to be above 95% by the gopan blue exclusion test.

Then, the experimental mice were inoculated subcutaneously or intraperitoneally through the right axillary, and each mouse was inoculated with 0.1mI cancer cell suspension, that is, 1×104 or 1×107 cancer cells.

4. Spleenectomy

Intraperitoneal anesthesia was used in combination with ketamine and phenobarbital, and the doses were 0.4 mg/10g and 0.2 mg/10g, respectively.

After anesthesia, the mouse was tied to a surgical board, the abdomen was clipped, iodine (2.5%) and alcohol (75%) were disinfected, and towels were spread. All layers of the abdominal wall were incised through the left lower abdomen and entered the abdominal cavity to expose the spleen and free it. Ligate the splenic pedicle with "0" silk thread and remove the spleen.

It is the strict aseptic operation during the operation, gentle movements, and thorough hemostasis.

During the operation, attention should be paid to whether there is an accessory spleen, and if there is, it should be removed together.

The control group simulated spleen incision, only incised the abdominal cavity and pulled the spleen, but did not remove it.

No antibiotics were used during or after surgery,

The incision infection rate was 1.0%, and the concentrate feeding was continued after the operation.

5. Preparation of spleen cell suspension and spleen tissue supernatant

1) Preparation of spleen cell suspension:

The newborn Kunming mice or adult mice that have just given birth for 24-48 hours are sacrificed, the abdominal wall is cut and the spleen is taken out, the spleen peripheral envelope and adipose tissue are cut off, and it is used in a non-bacterial glass plate.

Rinse the Han k's solution 3 times, then put the spleen into a glass homogenizer, add 5 ml of Han k's solution, grind the spleen tissue, filter with stainless steel wire mesh No. 100, centrifuge the filtrate (1000prm, 10min), and discard it. The clear solution was diluted with Hank's solution of the precipitated cells to prepare a 5×10^7/ml spleen cell suspension. The spleen cell survival rate was confirmed to be greater than 97% by staining with fetal pan blue. Then the spleen cell suspension was transplanted into the abdominal cavity of experimental mice. Each mouse only receives 2 mL of a spleen cell suspension from one recipient.

2) Preparation of spleen cell homogenate.

After the spleen is cut off, rapid freezing (-20^0C) and rapid rewarming are used to stain and microscopically confirm that there are no viable cells and the spleen cells have been lysed.

Then centrifuge the filtrate (1000 prm, 10min), save the supernatant, and discard the precipitate.

The supernatant was injected abdominally into the mice to be tested.

6. Observation items

1) Observe *the success rate* of cancer cell inoculation, the time of __appearance __ of subcutaneous tumor nodules and *the time or rate of tumor growth.*

2) Measure the diameter and size of subcutaneous tumor nodules with a caliper, measure the weight of mice, and observe metastasis and mobility.

3) Observe **the quality of life, coat color, vitality, nutritional status, breathing, mental status, and tumor-bearing survival period of tumor-bearing mice.**

4) It is to make ascite in the tumor-bearing mice, and tent to observe the shape and swelling degree of the abdomen.

According to the state of abdominal swelling, the amount of ascites is classified as 5 levels:

Grade 0: The abdomen is not full and there is no ascites formation, recorded as (1)

Grade 1: The abdomen is slightly raised with a small amount of ascites, recorded as (+)

Grade 2: Abdominal bulge, moderate ascites, recorded as (++)

Group 3: The abdomen is obviously raised and there is more ascites, which is recorded as (+++)

Group 4: The abdomen was in the shape of a frog belly with a lot of ascites, which was recorded as (++++)

During the autopsy, the amount of ascites was measured, the morphology of cancer cells were examined under microscope, and the rate and content of viable cells were counted.

5) Determine **the immune function status of red blood cells** in tumor-bearing mice, and measure the C3b receptor rosette test, using a semi-quantitative method.

6) Autopsy and pathological biopsy:

Autopsy each dead experimental mouse to observe the tumor's size, weight, infiltration and metastasis, the morphological and structural involvement of various organs, measure the amount of ascites, and take the tumor tissue and the liver, spleen, thymus, lung and other organs for pathology Biopsy.

2. The experimental results and analysis

1. *The comparison and analysis of results after subcutaneous inoculation of 0. 1 x 104 low-dose Ehrlich ascites carcinoma in the right armpit*

(1) The comparison of tumor nodule appearance time (md) with different treatment methods (T test), see Table 7.

Table 7

The comparison of appearance time (D) of tumor nodules with different treatment methods (T test)

Group	Group I-A1 (control group with spleen)	Group II-A3 (inoculation group after spleen cut)	Group III- (spleen cut group after inoculation)	IV-A1 group (first cut spleen and then inoculate + spleen tissue supernatant)
Day	8	7*	8	9*

Note:

(1) *Compared with the IA1 group, P<0.05 has significant meaning;

(2) One mouse in the I-A1 group (with spleen exposure group) (accounting for 7. 6%) experimental mice did not form tumor nodules after inoculation with cancer cells, and could survive for a long time (that is, the survival period exceeded 90 days).

No tumor was found during anatomy, it was deemed as a failure of the vaccination, and no statistical treatment was performed.

In IV-A group (intraperitoneal injection of spleen tissue supernatant group), 3 small experimental mice (25%) also failed inoculation.

In Table 7 and the above groups, tumor nodules appeared earliest in the spleen-cut and then inoculated group (II-A1 group).

The spleen control group and the spleen supernatant injection group were later.

(2) The comparison of the largest diameters of tumor nodules on the 7th, 14th, and 20th days in each group of different treatment methods. See Table 8.

Table 8

The comparison of tumor nodule size of each group on the 7th, 14th and 20th day of subcutaneous inoculation of 0.1X104 cancer cells (maximum diameter mm)

Unit: Maximum diameter mm

Group	l-Al (Control group with spleen)	II-Al (Inoculation group after spleen cut)	III-A (spleen cut group after vaccination)	IV-Al (cut the spleen, then inoculate+ spleen supernatant group)
Day 7 0	3.3±0.48	0	0	<0.0
Day 14 11.43±5.99	14.46.2	11.8±7.45	8±4.33	<0.01
Day 20 18.92±9.98	21.12±8.28	19.7±5.98	1 3.89±7.63	<0.01

Note: The P values in the table are obtained from the analysis of variance (F test).

It can be seen from the results in the table that the spleen is cut first and then inoculated (group II-A1). The tumor appears first and grows fastest.

Before the 14th day, his tumor was the largest.

On the 20th day after vaccination, the control group (I-A1 group), II-A1 group (first cut the spleen and then the vaccination group). The tumor size in the spleen excision group (III-A group) after inoculation first tended to be the same, while the splenic supernatant injection group (IV-A1 group) had the smallest size.

It shows that in the early stage of tumor growth (within the 7th day), the spleen has an anti-tumor effect, while in the middle and late stages (the proposed middle stage of this group of experiments is 8-14 days after vaccination, and 14 days later is the late stage of the tumor), the spleen inhibits The tumor effect is weakened or disappeared.

We also observed that the tumor nodules in the spleen-cut group were often liquefied and necroticed and fell off on the 14th day after inoculation with cancer cells, causing the tumor volume to shrink, and some even wound healing. This phenomenon needs further observation.

(3) Comparison of the maximum diameter **of tumor nodules** on the 7th, 14th, and 20th days of different treatment methods. See table 8

Table 8

Comparison of the size of tumor nodules on the 7th, 14th, and 20th days of each group of 0.1X104 cancer cells subcutaneously inoculated (maximum diameter mm)

Unit: Maximum diameter mm

Group	l-A1 (control group with spleen)	II-A1 (inoculation group after spleen-cut)	III-A (spleen-cut group after vaccination)	IV-A1 (spleen-cut, then inoculation+ spleen clearing fluid group}	P
Day -70 3.3 2 0.48 0 0 <0.01					
Day 14! 1.43 ± 5.99 14.46.2 11.8 ± 7.45 8 = 4.33 <0.01					
Day 20 18.92 II 9.98 21.12 = 8.28 19.7 II 5.98 1 3.89 == 7.63 <0.01					

Note: The P values in the table are all obtained from the analysis of diameter variance ((F test).

It can be seen from the results in the table that in the group that the spleen was cut first and then inoculated (Group II-A1), the tumor appeared first and grew fastest. Before the 14th day, the tumor had the largest volume.

On the 20th day after inoculation, the tumor size in these three group such as the control group (I-A1 group), II-A1 group (first spleen-cut and then inoculated group), III-A group (first vaccinated and then spleen-cut group) tended to be the same.

The spleen supernatant injection group (IV-A1 group) has the smallest volume.

It shows that in the early stage of tumor growth (within the 7th day), the spleen has tumor-inhibiting effect, while the middle and late stages (the mid-term proposed in this experiment is 8-14 days after inoculation, and the advanced stage of tumor after 14 days),

The suppressing effect of spleen on tumor becomes weak or disappears.

__We also observed that liquefied necrosis and shedding of tumor nodules often occurred on the 14th day after inoculation of tumor cells in the spleen-excised group, shrinking__

the tumor volume, and even wound healing. How this phenomenon occurs remains to be observed.

(4) Comparison of the average survival time of each group of 0.1×10^6 cancer cells subcutaneously inoculated. See Table 9.

Table 9

The comparison of survival time (days) of each group

Group	Group l-A1 (the control group with spleen)	Group II-A (the group with inocula tion after spleen-resec tion)	Group III-A (the group with spleen-cutoff after inoculation)	IV-A1 (the group with inocula tion after spleen-cutoff+ cleared spleen supernatant)	P
x̄±SD	41.61±12.24	38.73±19.63	44.8±15.95	50±27.21	<0.05

Note: The P is obtained by F test.

It can be seen from Table 9 that the survival time of the I-A1, II-A1, and III-A groups is close to each other.

After T test, there is no difference between the three groups, P> 0.05.

The survival time of the spleen supernatant injection group was significantly longer than that of the other groups, p <0.05, there was a significant difference.

2. The analysis of the results of each group of 0.1 x 104 cancer cells inoculated intraperitoneally

We considered those as a failure of vaccination who didn't develop the ascites or tumor nodules after inoculating the tumor cell, and those who can survive for more than 90 days without necropsy and no tumors, indicating that the inoculated cancer cells are rejected by the body. ***That implies that the inoculated cancer cells are rejected by the body and no tumors have formed***.

(1) 0.1X104 cancer cells were inoculated intraperitoneally with no ascites in each group **for the comparison of the inoculation failure rate**, see Table 10 below.

Table 10
The comparison of vaccination failure rate in each group (T test)

Group	Group l-A2 (the control group with spleen)	Group II-A2 (the group with inoculation after spleen-resection)	IV-A2 (the group with inoculation after spleen-cutoff+ cleared spleen supernatant)
THE failure rate	26%	0	54%*

Note: **means compared with the control group,T test P<0.01, there are highly significant differences,

*Means P<0.05, there is a significant difference.

Table 10 shows the results:

After the spleen was cut first, the inoculation group formed ascites, and the failure rate was 0.

There were 26% and 54% of the spleen control group and the injection on the spleen.

It proves that the tumor grows easily after tumor inoculation in the aspleen. In other words, cutting the spleen promotes tumor growth.

On the contrary, injection of spleen cell supernatant has the effect of inhibiting tumor growth.

(2) The comparison of survival time of each group of 0.1X104 cancer cells inoculated intraperitoneally, see Table 11

Table 11
The comparison of survival time ($\bar{x}\pm SQ$) of each group ((F test)

Group	l-A2 (the control group with spleen)	II-A2 (group with cut spleen before inoculation)	IV-A2 (group with spleen-resection before inoculation ±spleen supernatant)	P
$\bar{x}\pm SQ$	51.46± 29. 35	35.6±18.93	57.6 ± 14. 85	<0.05

It can be seen from Table 11 that the average survival time of the cancer cell group after cutting the spleen was 35.6±18.33 days, while the average survival time of the spleen control group and the spleen supernatant injection group were 51.40±29.25 and 57.6±14.86, P<0.05. There are significant differences between the 3 groups.

Among the 3 groups, the survival period was the shortest in the spleen-cut and inoculation group. The survival time of the spleen group was long, and the survival time of the spleenless group was short.

It shows that after splenectomy, it can promote tumor growth and shorten the survival period of tumor-bearing mice, while the injection of cell supernatant has a tumor-inhibiting effect and prolongs the survival period of tumor-bearing mice.

3. The results of subcutaneous inoculation of 0 1 x104 cancer cells in each group

(1) For the comparison of **the appearance** time of subcutaneous tumor nodules in each group, see Table 12.

Table 12

The comparison of appearance time of subcutaneous tumor nodules in each group

Group	Group I-B1 (The control Group with spleen)	Group II-B1 (The group with inoculation after spleen resection)	Group III-B (The group with spleen resection after inoculation)	Group IV-B1 (the group with inoculation after spleen resection ±spleen supernatant	P
Md (day)	5.5	5	7.5	9	<0.05

In the IIIB group, the spleen was cut on the 7th day after inoculation, so it was in the same condition as the spleen control group (I-B1) after 7 days.

The table indicates that the subcutaneous tumor nodules in the spleen first group appeared slightly earlier than the other groups, while the IV-B1 group (fetal splenocyte transplantation) appeared significantly later than the other groups.

It shows that the splenectomy has the effect of promoting tumor growth, and the transplantation of fetal splenocytes has the effect of strengthening the inhibition of tumor growth.

(2) Comparison of the average maximum diameter of subcutaneous tumor nodules on the 7, 14, and 20 days after inoculation in each group, see Table 13.

Table 13
The comparison of the maximum diameter of tumor nodules on days 7, 14, and 20 in each group

The unit: mm

Group	I-Bl	II-Bl	III-Bl	IV-Bl	P
	(the control Group with Spleen)	(The group with Inoculation after spleen cut)	(the group with spleen resection After Inoculation)	(the group with spleen resection after inoculation ±spleen supernatant)	
Day	7 5.07±1.	847 10.88±5.	278 2.83 ±1	.948 3.0±1.	56 <0.01
Day 14	19.85±4. 598	21.12±5.3	20.3±6.07	11±5.69	<0.01
Day 20	30.9±7.87	24±7.86	25.25±4.77	16±4.95	<0.01

Note: The P position in the table is obtained from F inspection or F-test.

(3) The comparison of the average survival time of each group is shown in Table 14.

Table 14
The comparison of the average survival time (days) of each group (0.1×10^7 cancer cells inoculated subcutaneously)

Group	I-Bl	II-Bl	III-Bl	IV-Bl	P
	(the control Group with Spleen)	(The group with Inoculation after spleen cut)	(the group with spleen resection After Inoculation)	(the group with spleen resection after inoculation ±spleen supernatant)	
$\bar{x}$±SD	33.1±13.15	49.56±24.39	38.7±14. 45	50.75±19.30	<0.01

As can be seen from Tables 13 and 14, there are the control group with spleen (I-Bl), the group with spleen-cut first and then vaccination (II-Bl), and the group with first vaccination and then spleen-cut(III-B).

72

In 7 days after vaccination of theses 3 groups are, the average maximum diameter of tumor nodules are $\bar{x}$ (I-B1) =5.076 ±1.847mm, $\bar{x}$ (II-B1)=10.88±5,275mm, $\bar{x}$(III-B1)=2.83±1.948mm, p<o. 01.

There is a significant difference between them.

The tumor volume is the largest in those who cut the spleen first and then inoculate (II-B1).

At this time, it is the 7th day. In fact, I-B1 and III-B are in the spleen group, and the spleen is in the active stage of proliferation, while the Il-B1 group is the spleen-free group.

The tumor is smaller in the spleen group, and in the spleen-free group the tumor is large in size, suggesting that the spleen can inhibit tumor in the early stage or promote tumor growth after splenectomy.

On the 14th day after vaccination, the average maximum diameter (mm) of the spleen tumor nodules in the three groups were $\bar{x}$(I -B1) =19.85±4.598, $\bar{x}$(II-B1)=21.15±5.3 and $\bar{x}$(III-B)) = 20.5±6.07, P>0.05, the difference between each other disappeared.

By the 20th day after inoculation, the volume of the control group with spleen was larger than the other groups, and the maximum diameter was =30.9±7.87 (mm).

At this time, the spleen of the tumor-bearing mice was extremely atrophic and lost its anti-tumor effect.

We have observed in our experiments that from the 14th day after inoculation in the spleen-cut group, most of the tumors of the mice began to liquefy and necrosis, and some of the tumors ruptured and fell off, and the volume became smaller. As for why the tumors will be necrotic and ulcerated during this period, the reason is still unclear and needs further observation.

In summary, it can be seen that the spleen can inhibit the growth of the tumor in the early stage of the tumor. The tumor in the spleen group has a slower growth rate and a smaller tumor size.

In the late stage of the tumor, the tumor suppressor effect weakens or disappears, and the tumor size of each group Converge.

In addition, it can be seen from the table that the fetal mouse spleen cell group (IV-B1 group) grew significantly slower, smaller in size, and had a longer survival than other groups in the spleen-cut and then inoculated and then transplanted fetal mouse splenocytes group.

It is proved that transplantation of allogeneic fetal spleen cells has obvious anti-tumor effect.

4. The results of intraperitoneal inoculation of $0.1/10^7$ cancer cells in each group

(1) The comparison of ascites time in each group. See Table 15 for

Table 15

The comparison of the time (days) for the appearance of ascites in each group after intraperitoneal inoculation of 0.1×10^7 cancer cells

Group	I-B2	II-B2	IV-B1
	(the control Group with Spleen)	(the group with spleen resection After Inoculation)	(the group with spleen resection after inoculation ±spleen supernatant)
Means	5	3*	4*

Note: **there is significant while compared with control group, T test P<0.05

(2) 0.1×107 cancer cells were inoculated into each group on the 5th, 7th and 14th day of ascites greater than (++), the percentage ratio, see Table 16.

Table 16

The comparison of the amount of ascites with 0.1×107 cancer cells inoculation in abdominal cavity

Day of inoculation	I-B2 (the control Group with Spleen)	II-B2 (the group with spleen resection After Inoculation)	IV-B1 (the group with spleen resection after inoculation ±spleen supernatant)
2	0%	75%	10%
7	28%	100%	70%
14	100%	100%	100%

Note: *means I-B2 (control group) comparison, T test P<0.01, * means P<0.05, no *means P>0.05

(3) The survival time of each group inoculated with 0.1×10^7 cancer cells through the abdomen (days)

Group	I-B2 (the control Group with Spleen)	II-B2 (the group with spleen resection After Inoculation)	IV-B1 (the group with spleen resection after inoculation ±spleen supernatant
$\bar{x} \pm SD$	20.15±4.59	15.56± 10.94*	16.67 ±8.34

Note:

It means that compared with I-B2 group, P<0.05 is significant difference;

It means that compared with I-B1 group, F>0.05 has no significant difference,

Combining the results in Tables 15, 16, and 17, these results suggest that the first spleenectomy group (II-B2) has a faster tumor growth rate, more ascites, shorter survival period, and easy to find organ metastasis, indicating that the splenectomy has the effect of promoting tumor growth.

Transplantation of allogeneic adult mouse spleen cells through the abdomen can partially inhibit tumor growth, but the tumor suppression effect is weaker than that of the spleen control group, and is not as good as that of transplanted fetal spleen cells. In another word, the allogeneic adult mouse spleen cells can partially inhibit tumor growth, but the tumor suppression effect is weaker than that of the spleen control group, and it is not as good as the **transplanted fetal spleen cell.**

5. Autopsy and pathological examination results

Each mouse was autopsied after death, the shape of the tumor, the involvement of the organs and the spread of the tumor were observed with naked eyes, and the tissues were taken for pathological examination.

The result prompts:

The Ehrlich ascites cancer strain has the characteristics of stable proliferation and migration, strong invasiveness, etc. It is easy to form solid tumors by subcutaneous inoculation.

Autopsy confirmed that tumors or ascites were easily formed locally after inoculation, and the surrounding tissues were easily infiltrated.

Subcutaneously vaccinated patients have less metastasis, while intraperitoneal vaccinated patients are more likely to have **liver, kidney, and lymph node metastasis in the late stage.**

Only 2 of the 270 experimental mice had splenic metastases, suggesting that the spleen itself has a low affinity for cancer.

This group of experiments also found that in the spleen first and then intraperitoneal inoculation group, multiple cancer metastases were found in the abdominal organs, and the metastasis rate was found to reach 50%, mainly **involving the liver, kidney, pancreas and mesenteric lymph nodes, and often involving more than 2 organs.**

The spleen control group and the allogeneic spleen cell transplantation group had fewer metastases. The metastasis rates were 20% and 25%, which were significantly lower than those in the without spleen group.

It indicates that the spleen can inhibit the growth of tumors, but the asplenic group loses the tumor-inhibiting effect, which leads to the easy spread of tumors.

In addition, during the dynamic observation of the experimental mice in this group, it was found that the thymus and spleen of the tumor-bearing mice undergo a series of changes with the progression of the disease, and there is a certain regularity.

About 7 days after inoculation, the thymus showed acute progressive atrophy, and the volume decreased, from a normal leaflet diameter of 5--8 cm to about 1mm; the weight decreased from 70 ± 10 mg to 20 ± 5 mg, while the spleen was Immediately after inoculation of cancer, hyperemia, swelling, volume increase, weight increase, texture becomes brittle, germinal centers increase under microscopy, cell proliferation is active, and the spleen rapidly shrinks and shrinks in size at the 14th largest after inoculation, the weight is reduced from 140 ± 15 mg to 50 ± 10 mg, the germinal center is significantly reduced, cell proliferation is blocked, accompanied by fibrous tissue hyperplasia, fibrosis, the color is gray, and the texture becomes hard.

6. Measurement results of red blood cell immune function

In this group of experiments, 100 mice were tested for red blood cell c3b receptor rosette.

The results suggest that the c3b receptor rosette binding rate of tumor-bearing mice showed a progressive decline after splenectomy. It shows that the immune adhesion ability of red blood cells decreased after spleen cut

3. Discussion

1. ***It can be seen from the experimental results that the spleen has the effect of inhibiting tumor growth or that*** the spleen can inhibit tumor growth

After spleenectomy, tumor growth was faster than that of the control group, and the appearance of subcutaneous tumor nodules was earlier than that of the control group.

During the same period, the volume of subcutaneous tumor nodules was also larger.

In the intraperitoneal inoculation group with cancer cells, ascites appeared earlier and the volume of ascites was also larger in the spleenectomy group.

The content of cancer cells is also higher, and the survival period is shorter than that of the control group with spleen.

Autopsy revealed that the metastasis rate of cancer in the spleen excised group was higher than that in the control group, about 30% (liver, kidney, pancreas, mesenteric lymph node metastasis).

It can be seen from Table 13 that the two groups of II-B2 (first cut the spleen and then vaccination group) and IIIB (first cut the spleen after vaccination) have the spleen cut at different times.

On the 7th day after inoculation, the average maximum diameters of the subcutaneous tumor nodules were II-B1$\bar{x}$=10.8±5.28 and IIIBX=2.83±1.845, respectively, the former was significantly larger than the latter.

However, on the 14th day after vaccination, the tumors in group IIIB proliferated rapidly after spleenectomy, and the difference between the two quickly disappeared, IIIB1$\bar{x}$ = 21.2 ± 5.3, II-B$\bar{x}$ = 20.3 ± 6.07, P>0.05, there was no significant difference.

It is suggested that the removal of the spleen can promote tumor growth, in other words, the spleen can inhibit tumor growth.

In the past 20 years, it has been discovered that the spleen not only plays a great role in fighting infections, but also plays an important role in anti-tumor immunity.

The mechanism of action may be through the production of NK cells, macrophages (Mφ), LAK cells, TH/Ti cells, B cells, Ts cells and other cellular immune functions and the secretion of Tufisn factor, TNF factor, IL-2, interferon, Complement, antibodies and other lymphokines to kill tumor cells,

Ge Yigong once used the rat Lw56 lung sarcoma model to investigate the effect of spleen cut on tumor growth.

It is believed that the success rate of tumor inoculation after spleen incision is higher than that of the spleen group, and the metastasis rate is increased, similar to the experimental results of this group.

The experimental results of this group also indicate that after splenectomy, the binding rate of c3b receptor rosette in peripheral blood of the body decreased by 40% compared with the healthy group with spleen, indicating that the body's red blood cell immune function decreased after splenectomy.

2. ***The inhibitory effect of the spleen on tumor growth mainly occurs in the early stage of the tumor, and in the late stage of the tumor, the inhibitory effect of the spleen on tumor growth weakens or disappears***

It can be seen from Table 8 and Table 13 that in the early stage of the tumor (7 days), the spleen-cut group had a faster tumor growth than the spleen control group. The subcutaneous tumor nodules are large in size and have a lot of ascites.

In the advanced stage of the tumor (14 days later), the volume of tumor nodules in the spleen control group and the spleen cut group was basically the same, which was not significantly comparable.

There is no significant difference in survival time.

We performed autopsy and disease examination on 300 experimental mice and found that the spleen of tumor-bearing mice had some regular changes as the disease progressed.

In the early stage of tumor development (within 7days after the inoculation of cancer cells), **because of the tumor cell stimulation, the spleen has congestion and swelling of the spleen, increased volume, accelerated cell proliferation, and increased germinal center**s.

In the late stage of the tumor (from the 14th day after vaccination), the spleen showed progressive atrophy, shrinking in size, sharply reduced germinal centers, and fibrous tissue proliferation.

It was found that there is splenic fibrosis. As a result, its anti-cancer immune effect is weakened or disappeared.

It is even possible to suppress the body's anti-cancer immunity and promote tumor growth through suppressive T cells, macrophages and immunosuppressive factors.

It shows that the spleen has a two-way effect on the immune status of tumors, and has obvious timing, which is related to the disease stage of the tumor.

The early spleen shows anti-tumor effect, and the late stage shows immunosuppressive effect.

However, the root cause of the immunosuppressive state of the body is the tumor itself, and the spleen only plays a certain role in the formation of this state.

3. *Intraperitoneal injection of healthy splenocyte supernatant and transplantation of allogeneic splenocytes can inhibit tumor growth*

Compared with the other groups, the spleen cell supernatant injection or spleen cell transplantation group (IV group) showed that the tumor growth in this group was slower than other groups, the tumor nodules appeared later, the volume was smaller, and the amount of ascites was less.

After a small dose of 0.1X104 cancer cells were inoculated, the success rate of tumor-bearing mice was significantly lower than that of other groups.

In addition, a few small fluoride first appeared with oligohuang ascites or small subcutaneous tumor nodules, *the tumor can disappear naturally, and the survival period is more than 90 days (as long-term survival).*

Among them, the anti-tumor effect of transplanted allogeneic fetal spleen cells (IV-B1 **group) is particularly significant, with a tumor suppression rate of 54%, and a survival period of 17 days longer than the control group.**

The disease examination of this group of tumor-bearing mice found that after transplantation of allogeneic fetal spleen cells, 7 mice (accounting for 50%) had splenic islands formed in the abdominal cavity or (and) mesentery.

These spleen cells have the characteristics of weak antigenicity, small amount, and strong cell proliferation.

After allogeneic transplantation, it is not easy to produce a strong rejection reaction, and it is not restricted by ABO blood type, and there is no need for blood type cross test.

Some people in China use **traumatic spleen cells to prepare LAK cells to treat advanced malignant tumors and obtain better curative effects, which can inhibit tumor growth and prolong life.**

At present, adoptive immunotherapy with fetal spleen cell transplantation has not been reported in the literature.

This group of experiments needs further discussion.

4. *The body's anti-tumor immunity is negatively correlated with the number of cancer cells*

This group of experiments found that the body's anti-tumor immune effect is significantly affected by the number of cancer cells inoculated.

If the number of cancer cells is small, the anti-tumor effect will be stronger and more pronounced.

On the contrary, the anti-tumor effect will be very weak.

For example, if a person is inoculated with 0.1×10^7 cancer cells, the immune function of the body will be significantly suppressed.

There was a big difference in the tumor growth rate between the spleen-cut group and the spleen group in the early stage, and after the middle stage (7 days later), the difference quickly disappeared, and there was no significant difference in survival.

However, if the group was inoculated with 0.1×10^4 cancer cells, the body's anti-tumor effect became more prominent.

The inoculation failure rate with spleen tissue was significantly higher than that in the without spleen group, the tumor grew slowly, the nodule size was small, and the survival time was longer.

In addition, the tumor suppressor immune enhancement effect after transplantation of allogeneic spleen cells in the low-dose cancer cell group was also obvious, the tumor growth rate was significantly slowed, and some tumor nodules could even disappear naturally after formation and survive for a long time.

This result indicates that the body's anti-tumor effect is negatively related to the number of inoculated cancer cells.

However, the immunosuppressive effect of cancer on the body is positively correlated with the number of inoculated cancer cells.

The spleen is involved in the regulation of tumor immunity and has a dual effect on the immune status of tumor-bearing mice, and it exhibits a certain anti-tumor effect in the early stage.

As the tumor develops, the number of tumor cells increases, and the spleen gradually shrinks, which turns into an immunosuppressive effect.

But the basic cause of the immunosuppressive state is the tumor itself.

As the cancer progresses, the number of cancer cells increases and the inhibitory effect is strengthened, leading to atrophy of immune organs such as the spleen and thymus.

5. *The results of this group of experiments prompted*

(1) The spleen has a certain anti-tumor effect. In the early stage of the tumor, it can inhibit the growth of the tumor. At the later stage of the disease, the anti-tumor effect of the spleen weakens or disappears, and may even promote the growth of the tumor.

(2) Adoptive immunity after transplantation of allogeneic fetal spleen cells can strengthen the body's immune and anti-cancer effects and inhibit tumor growth.

(3) The body's anti-cancer immune effect is negatively correlated with the number of tumor cells. The more cancer cells there are, the more easily the immune function of the body is inhibited or damaged. The faster the tumor grows, the worse the prognosis.

9

The article Four

The experimental study on combined transplantation of fetal liver, fetal spleen and fetal thymus cells for adoptive immune reconstruction to treating malignant tumors

One

The experimental study on adoptive immunoreconstruction through combined transplantation of fetal liver, fetal spleen and fetal thymus cells for treatment of malignant tumors

In this paper, the same kind of the transplantation of fetal liver, fetal spleen, and fetal thymocytes were used on Ehrlich ascites carcinoma (EAC) subcutaneous solid tumor type mice for systematic adoptive immune reconstruction to treatming malignant tumor. And it was set up a single fetal liver, fetal spleen, fetal thymus cell transplantation and the combination of fetal liver cell + fetal spleen cell, fetal liver cell + fetal thymus cell, fetal spleen paper cell + fetal thymus cell transplantation group for double transplantation treatment group. The tumor growth, regression, survival time, cellular immune indicators and various histopathological examinations were systematically observed to compare the efficacy of each group in mice or /and the efficacy of each group was compared.

The results showed that the difference in efficacy was in the order of triple group> double group> single cell transplantation group.

In the triple cell transplantation treatment group, the complete tumor regression rates in the near and long-term observation groups were 40% (n = 15) and 46.67% (n = 15), and the partial regression rates (tumor regression> 50%) reached 26.67% and

13.33%. The rat patients with complete tumor regression have long-term survival, and partial regression has an average survival time of more than 1 month.

The immune index has improved significantly, and the immune organs are hypertrophic. Tissue sections or slices of <u>immune organs</u> show that **the cells proliferate actively**. Pathological sections of the <u>tumor tissue</u> showed that **a large number of lymphocytes infiltrated around the tumor tissue and in the interstitium to form a package, and the central tumor tissue showed pathological phenomena such as coagulation, liquefaction necrosis and nuclear fragmentation.**

In the dual cell transplantation treatment group, there was no complete regression except for a few cases of partial regression.

Immunological indicators improved, prolonged survival and lymphocyte infiltration of tumor tissue were not as good as those of triple cell transplantation treatment group.

The tumor regression, survival period, immune index improvement and pathological examination results <u>of the single cell transplantation</u> treatment group were not as obvious as those of the first two, but were superior to the tumor-bearing control group.

It shows that the system adoptive immune reconstruction can **better** anti-tumor immune function and improve the curative effect through the overall synergy of the system than the partial reconstruction.

With the introduction of biological response regulation theory (BRM), a profound revolution is taking place in the field of tumor therapy. The fourth-generation tumor treatment program-tumor biotherapy has become the focus of attention in the field of tumor treatment after surgery, chemotherapy, and radiotherapy. **A large number of clinical and experimental studies have found that with the progression of the tumor stage, the body's immune status shows progressive suppression.**

<u>How to restore and rebuild the anti-tumor immune function of the tumor-bearing body is the core of tumor biotherapy research.</u>

Adoptive immunotherapy with Rosenberg as the representative has made outstanding achievements in this field.

In addition to the transfer of immunocompetent cells expanded in vitro and artificially obtained various immune factors, adoptive immunotherapy, ***<u>embryonic-derived immune organs and cell transplantation are another promising research content</u>***.

China has a wide range of embryo sources. This technology of the expensive biological therapy has the advantages of economy, simple technology and easy promotion. It is a direction worthy of in-depth research and exploration.

In recent years, many domestic authors have successively carried out research on the transplantation of **embryonic liver, spleen, and thymus from cells, tissue blocks** to organ levels for the treatment of advanced malignant tumors, and have achieved certain results.

With the in-depth study of the immune system, the source, proliferation, differentiation and function of lymphocytes, as well as the function and role of the middle-structured immune organs and peripheral immune organ tubes in the immune response have been basically understood.

At present, when adopting embryonic-derived immune organ transplantation for adoptive immunotherapy of tumors, most of them use single embryonic organs, such as fetal liver cell transplantation, fetal spleen, thymus cell transplantation, and tissue slice transplantation. Whether adoptive reconstruction can be carried out from the overall level of the system, that is, simultaneous reconstruction of central immunity and peripheral immunity to improve the efficacy, there is no similar literature in the world.

Combined fetal liver, spleen, and thymocyte transplantation, which includes fetal liver cell transplantation, has the function of bone **marrow transplantation**, and **combined fetal thymus and spleen cell transplantation can make immune adoptive reconstruction** close to the establishment of the overall system level. Can it play a synergistic role? Improve treatment is worth exploring and research.

(1) Materials and methods

1. *Animal and tumor models*

(1) Experimental animals:

In a closed group, there were 200 Kunming mice, 5-6 weeks old, weighing 18 ± 2.1g, male or female.

(2) Tumor model equipment:

After the recovery of EhrlIch ascites carcinoma cell strain, prepare ascites type rats. After the ascites are formed, extract the ascites of cancer cells and wash them 3 times with Hank's solution (800rpm), 5 minutes each time, discard the supernatant, adjust the precipitated cancer cells Hank's solution The cell concentration is up to 10 ml. It has been confirmed by the Eosin rejection test that the viable cell rate is> 95%.

The right mouse intestine was subcutaneously seeded with 0.1 ml / mouse. After 1 week, all tumor nodules with a diameter of d = 9.5 + 1.5 mm appeared under the skin of the inoculation site, and a model of Ehrlich-bearing ascites carcinoma subcutaneous solid tumor was developed.

2. *The experimental grouping*

The experimental animals were randomly divided into tumor-bearing control groups (group B, n = 9);

The long-term observation group (Cl group, n = 15) and the short-term observation group (CII group) of fetal liver, spleen, and thymocytes combined transplantation treatment were treated with combined cell transplantation once a week, and were killed after 5 consecutive times, n = 15);

Fetal liver cell transplantation treatment group (group F);

Fetal spleen cell transplantation treatment group (group G);

Fetal thymus cell transplantation treatment group (group H);

Fetal liver and spleen cells combined transplantation treatment group (group I);

Fetal liver and thymus cells combined transplantation treatment group ((group K);

nF = nG = nH = nJ = nK = 12.

After successful modeling, each group underwent corresponding cell transplantation once a week, and observed after 5 consecutive times.

3. *The preparation of fetal liver, spleen, thoracic and spleen cell suspension*

Take the stage to pair the pregnant females with 15-18 days of gestation, and take the fetuses by aseptic laparotomy.

The liver, spleen, and thymus were separated and rinsed in sterile Han k's solution at 4 ° C, and then homogenized in sterile tissue homogenate, diluted with 4C Hank's solution, filtered, and the cell-rich suspension was collected. Sampling for bacterial culture and pyrogen test are both negative and used for separate equipment.

4. *The ways and methods of cell transplantation*

Fetal liver cell transplantation:

Take 0.2m of the prepared hepatocyte suspension and inject it into the tail vein;

Fetal spleen cell transplantation:

Take the prepared spleen cell suspension 0.2m / piece / time and inject it intraperitoneally,

Fetal thymus cell transplantation:

Take the prepared thymus cell suspension 0.2mt / piece / time and intramuscular injection in the hind leg.

In each experiment, treatment was started one week after the inoculation of cancer cells, once a week for 5 consecutive times, and the control group was treated with the same amount of Han k's solution as the control treatment.

5. *The items for the Observation:*

(1) The general items:

After inoculation of tumor cells, observe the time of tumor appearance, and measure the size of tumor nodules (average vertical diameter 2) with a vernier caliper every other day, quality of life of mice, tumor growth and survival time (days).

(2) The dynamic observation of peripheral blood T lymphocyte count:

In this experiment, a-acetate acetate staining method was used to determine the peripheral blood lymphocytes (ANAE).

First prepare hexaazo by-pin red solution and 2% a-acetate tea cool enzyme solution, store in 4 C protected from light for future use.

Before use, take 89ml of phosphate buffer solution of 1 / 15mol / l, PH value of 7.6, slowly add 6ml of hexaazo by-pin red solution, mix well, then slowly add 2.5ml of 2% a-acetate tea incubation enzyme solution, fully Mix well, and finally make amber bluff color sample solution, PH value to 6.4 to make an incubation solution, immerse the incubation solution in a 37 ° C water bath to preheat.

Cut off 0.2mm of the tail of the mouse, take the blood piece, dry it in natural wind and immerse it in the incubation solution for 1-3 hours, rinse it with tap water, dry it, add 1% methyl green dye solution for 1-3 minutes, and wash it with tap water After drying,

Observed by oil microscope, the black-red particles (generally 2-5) with different sizes and numbers in the cytoplasm are ANAE positive cells.

Count 200 lymphocytes and calculate the percentage of T lymphocytes. They were measured 1 week after model building, 1 week after treatment, and 1 week apart thereafter, and were dynamically observed.

(3) The dynamic observation of lymphocyte transformation rate:

The morphological method was used to detect the whole blood in vitro.

First prepare complete RP-M1640 medium (1640 is a product of the Japanese Strain Society, each bag contains 1640 powder 10.4g), which contains inactivated calf serum 20%, 30.0g / L L-glutamine 1ml, sterilized 60.0 g / L NaHCO3 3ml, penicillin 10000u, streptavidin 10000ug.

Strictly disinfect the rat tail, cut off the tail 0.2mm, use sterile heparinized micro sampler to collect 0.1ml blood, add 1.8ml complete medium, then add 0.1ml PHA, Incubate in a 37'C constant temperature water-isolated incubator for 72 hours, shaking once a day.

At the end of the incubation period, remove most of the supernatant, add 8.5g / L NH4CL 4ml, mix and place in a 37 ° C water bath for 10 minutes, centrifuge at 2500rpm for 10 minutes, discard the supernatant, add 5ml of fixed solution (9 parts of methanol, ice-cold) 1 part of acid), centrifuge at room temperature for 10 minutes, discard the supernatant (1500rpm for 5 minutes), add Hanks solution to 0.2ml of the precipitate, mix well and drop it on clean glass slides to make it spread evenly.

Giemsa staining solution was stained for 5 minutes, washed with tap water, and after drying, 200 lymphocytes were observed under an oil microscope to calculate the conversion rate of blasts.

The **same T cell counts were also measured 1 week after modeling, 1 week after the start of** treatment, and every other week thereafter, and observed dynamically.

(4) Determination of wet weight of immune organs

Carry out a thorough and thorough necropsy on all dead and sacrificed experimental mice, completely cut out the thymus and spleen, observe the size, weigh them with a torque balance, and calculate the wet weight (mg) / weight (g) of the immune organs of each mouse.

(5) Pathological examination

All the dead and killed rats were systematically pathologically dissected to observe the tumor infiltration and metastasis. *The tumor tissue, thymus, spleen, lung, liver, kidney and other organs were taken for a slice of tissue disease, and focus on the observation of lymphocyte infiltration in tumor tissue and pathological changes of immune organs.*

(2) The experimental results

1. The comparison of the average survival time (geometric mean method) of mice in each group and the survival rate of different tumor ages:

It can be seen from Table 1 that the survival time of each treatment group is significantly longer than that of the control group, P <0.05, especially in the triple cell transplantation treatment group, P <0.01. There is also a significant difference between the three treatment groups in other treatment groups, P <o.o5.

<u>Seven tumors in the CI group completely regressed and achieved long-term survival without tumor recurrence.</u>

Two cases of tumors regressed> 50%. After 2 months of survival, they relapsed and died.

Table 1 The comparison of the survival time in each group
and the survival rate in the different age rats

Group	N	The survived time(d) ($\bar{x}$+SEM)	the survival rate with the different survival times(%)							
			1(Week)	2(week)	3(week)	4(week)	5(week)	6(week)	2(month)	3(month)
B group	9	13.3 ± 1.3	100	55.6	11.1	11.1	0	0	0	0
F group	12	* 22.5± 1.6**	100	83. 3	58. 3*	50	33.3	33.3	0**	0**
G group	12	*21.4 ±1.9**	100	75	66. 7*	50	33. 3	16.7**	0**	0**
H group	12	*26.2±1.4**	100	100	75*	58.3*	41.7	33. 3	0**	0**
I group	12	*27.4±1.7**	100	91. 7	66.7*	50	33.3	33.3	8.3**	0 **
J group	12	*28.3 ± 1.8**	100	83.3	3.75*	66.7*	41.7	41.7	16.7	0**
K group	12	*23 ± 1.5**	100	100	75*	58.3*	41.7	25	16.7	0**
CI group	15	47.2 ± 2.0°	100	93. 3	80*	73.3*	66. 7*	60*	46.7*	46.7*

Note:

1. B in the table is the tumor-bearing control group:

F is the fetal liver cell treatment group;

G is the fetal spleen cell treatment group:

H is the fetal thymus cell treatment group;

I is the fetal liver and spleen cell group;

J is the fetal liver + thymus cell group:

K is the fetal thymus + spleen cell group;

CI is fetal liver + spleen+ thymus cell group

2. In the table :

* P <0.05 for each treatment group and control group; Compare with the control group P<0.01;

°Comparison of treatment group with CI group P <0.05;

** treatment group with Cl group p <0.01

From the perspective of survival rates at different tumor ages, at the third week of tumor bearing, each treatment group showed significant differences compared with the control group.

With the extension of the disease period and the extension of the observation period, the Cl group and the control group always showed significant differences, while the other treatment groups gradually lost the difference compared with the control group, and showed significant differences with the CI group.

2. Treatment and efficacy analysis See table 2

Table 2 The analysis of the efficacy of each group

Group	N	cured rate	significant effective rate	having effective rate	invalid	total effective rate
Group B	90	0$^{\triangle\triangle}$	0	0	100	0
Group F	12	0$^{\triangle\triangle}$	0	34.4 (4)	66.4 (8)	33.4 (4)$^{\triangle\triangle}$
Group G	12	0$^{\triangle\triangle}$	0	25 (3)	75 (9)	25 (3) $^{\triangle\triangle}$
Group H	12	0$^{\triangle\triangle}$	8.3 (1)	33.4 (4)	58.3 (7)	41.7 (5)*
Group I	12	0$^{\triangle\triangle}$	8.3 (1)	33.4(4)	58.3 (7)	41.7 (5)$^{*\triangle}$
Group J	12	0$^{\triangle\triangle}$	26.67 (2)	41.7 (5)	41.7 (5)	58.3 (7)
Group K	12	0$^{\triangle\triangle}$	26. 67 (2)	33.4 (4)	50 (6)	50 (6)*
CI Group	15	46.7**	13. 3 (2)	20 (3)	20 (3)	80 (12)**

Note:
* Indicates comparison with control group P <0.05,
** P <0.01 compared with the control;
$\triangle$ indicates P <0.05 compared with CI,
$\triangle\triangle$ indicates P <0.01 compared with CI

The efficacy criteria:

① The cure:
The tumor completely regressed and achieved long-term survival without tumor recurrence;

② Significant effect:
Part of the tumor regressed significantly (regression> 50%), and the survival period was more than 2 months;

③ Effective:
The survival time was more than doubled, and the tumor did not regress significantly.

④ Invalid:
The tumor grows progressively and dies within a short period (3-4 weeks).

As can be seen from Table 2, the cure rate of the CI group was 46.67%, which was very significant compared with the other groups, p <0.01.

There was no significant difference between the groups in the apparent efficiency and effective efficiency.

The comparison of total efficiency suggests that, except for the single hepatocyte spleen cell treatment group, the total effective rates of the other treatment groups are significantly different from those of the control group, and the difference in efficacy is triple> double> single.

In addition, **in the single-cell transplantation group, the TH cell group had the best efficacy, and the TH cell group had a higher efficacy than the non-TH cell group in the dual cell transplantation cells.**

It shows **that thymus cells play a key role in this treatment process**; the single liver and spleen vascular transplantation has little effect, and the combination of two can improve the efficacy, and the combination of the three can significantly improve the efficacy.

3. The observation and comparison of tumor growth rate and regression prognosis

In this experiment, a pseudo-clinical method was used to establish medical records for each group of experimental rats, and the tumor growth rate, regression and prognosis of each experimental mouse were recorded in detail.

The vernier ruler was used to measure the average vertical diameter of the tumor every other day, and the final measured value of all death cases was used as the calculated value of the effective sample parameter in each subsequent measurement in the same group.

One week after modeling, the tumor grew rapidly, with an average vertical diameter of 9.5 ± 1.5mm,

One week after the start of treatment, the tumor continued to grow, and by the second week after the start of treatment, the groups showed differences, the tumor in the control group still grew rapidly, and the tumor-bearing mice progressively failed.

All died within 4 weeks, single-cell transplanted tumors grew slowly, and the quality of life was significantly improved. All tumor-bearing mice died within 2 months.

In the two-cell transplantation group, the tumor growth was significantly inhibited. Among them, 5 cases showed significant partial regression, and all tumor-bearing mice died within 3 months.

Nine patients in the triple cell transplantation group had obvious tumor necrosis and ulceration.

Among them, 7 cases completely regressed within 5-6 weeks, and the ulcers were cured, and 2 cases regressed by more than 50%. Except for 2 cases that died at 2 and 3 weeks, the tumor growth was stagnant until Failure and death.

Seven cases with complete tumor regression achieved long-term survival without tumor recurrence. So far, it has been more than 6 months and has normal pregnancy and delivery capabilities. From the above observations, it can be found that single or dual cell transplantation has the functions of inhibiting tumor growth, improving quality of life, and prolonging survival.

Triple cell transplantation not only inhibits tumor growth but may also cause significant tumor regression or partial regression and prolonged survival.

4. Dynamic observation of peripheral blood T lymphocyte count and lymphocyte transformation rate

According to the results in Table 3 and Table 4, the cell immune index of each experimental group was significantly lower than that of normal mice 1 week after modeling, with an average decrease of more than 50% (normal group T cell count X = 62.5 ± 1.7, Lymphatic transfer X = 66.8 ± 4.8), indicating that the development of tumors suppresses immune function.

One week after the start of treatment, the immune index system of each treatment group and the control group and after treatment and before treatment were significantly improved (P <O.05), and there was no significant difference between the treatment groups.

Looking at the growth of the tumor, at this time, although there is an improvement in the immune index system, there is no obvious tumor suppressing effect.

Continued dynamic observation showed that after each group of single cell transplantation and dual cell transplantation, tumor growth inhibition and immune index improvement continued for a period of time (about 3 to 4 weeks), the immune index system tended to decline, and the disease of tumor-bearing mice also followed deterioration.

This is consistent with reports of clinical monitoring of tumor patients' immune function to judge prognosis.

The immune index of the dual cell transplantation group continued to improve, especially in cases of tumor regression.

The long-term surviving cases are still close to normal mice after 2 months.

For those whose condition is getting worse, the above indicators are measured before death, and they have dropped to below the pre-treatment level.

It shows that the cellular immune index is indeed a good evidence to reflect the efficacy and judge the prognosis,

It also indirectly proves that embryonic-derived immune cell transplantation can indeed achieve the purpose of rebuilding the immune function of tumor-bearing bodies.

Table 3

The dynamic observation table of the peripheral blood T lymphocyte count (ANAE)

Group	N	T lymphocyte count ($\bar{x}$±SEM)							
		n	1W	n	2W	n	4W	n	6W
Group B	9	9	3.42±4.8	5	29.1±2.9	1	32	0	
Group F	12	12	31.4±3.6	10	54.6±5.12*△	6	48.7±2.2	4	36.7± 4.9
Group G	12	12	35.5±3.9	9	52.5±4.7*△	6	46.6±3.3	2	33.4±5.1
GroupH	12	12	32.6±4.1	12	56.6±4.1	7	50.9±2.1	4	40.7±3.8
GroupI	12	12	36.2±2.7	11	53.4±3.5	6	55.3±3.6	4	39.3±4.2
GroupJ	12	12	30.8±4.3	10	55.8±3.8	8	56.4±1.9	5	42.6±2.7
GroupK	12	12	33.7±3.4	12	57.3±4.4	7	55.8±2.8	3	41.3±4.5
CI group	15	15	31.8 ± 3.	:,,	59. 6 ± 2. 6	mutual,	62.5 ± '7"	9	67.8 ± 34 △

Note:

* indicates comparison with the control group $P < 0.05$.

△ indicates that $P < 0.05$ was compared after the treatment started and before the treatment.

Table 4

The dynamic observation of peripheral blood lymphocyte transformation rate

Group	N		Lymphocyte transformation rate ($\bar{x}\pm$SEM)						
		n	1W	n	2W	n	4W	n	6W
Group B	9	9	3.25 ± 5.4	5	25.51 ± 3.6	1	28	0	
Group F	2	12	31.6±3.7	10	51.2±2.7°△	6	54.2±6.1△	4	36.1±5.4
Group G	12	12	29.8±4.3	9	48.4±4.6°△	6	52.8±1.8*	2	33.6±2.5
GroupH	12	12	34.1±4.1	12	56.6±2.1°△	7	52.4±3.7△	4	40.7±1.9△
GroupI	12	12	28.5±5.1	11	53.4±3.5°△	6	50.5±2.9△	4	37.3±3.2△
GroupJ	12	12	29.4 ± 2.9	10	58.1±3.5°△	8	60.6±3.4△	5	46.5 ± 6△
GroupK	12	12	30.7±1.8	12	54.9±5.2°△	7	57.5 ± 4.3△	3	45.8 ± 3.9△
Group CI	15	15	31.5±3.2	14	55.8±2.8°△	11	63. 9±3.2△	9	66.8±4.8△

Note:

* indicates comparison with Group comparison $p < 0.05$:

△ indicates that after the start of treatment and before treatment $P < 0.05$

5. Anatomical observation of immune organs and comparative analysis of wet weight of immune organs

See Table 5 and Table 6.

In order to understand the changes in the immune organs of tumor-bearing organisms and their correlation **with the efficacy,** we also set up a recent observation group of triple cell transplantation (CII group, n = 15, of which 6 tumors completely regressed and 4 cases regressed> 50%). After the model was treated with the CII group for 5 times, all were executed. At the same time, a normal control group was set up, and Hank's solution was used for simulated modeling and control treatment.

It is to observe the changes of immune organs anatomically, to weigh the wet weight of immune organs, to calculate the ratio of immune organs to body weight, and to compare with other experimental groups.

As a result, it was found that in all experimental groups, the **thymus of all cases of progressive tumor death was significantly atrophy, and the degree of atrophy was positively correlated with tumor progression.** The atrophied thymus is dull in color and extremely brittle in quality. The spleen is less obvious than the thymus. Most of them showed changes in congestion and swelling, and a few showed changes in atrophy. However, **in the CII group, where the tumor completely resolved or significantly regressed, the thymus and spleen showed significant hypertrophy, and the thymus index and spleen index increased**. Not only is there a significant difference between the death cases of each group (or cases of tumor without regression), but also a significant difference from the normal control group.

Table 5

Comparison of the wet weight of immune organs in each group within 6 weeks of death and normal control group

Group	N	Thymus (mg) / body weight (g) X± SEM	Spleen (mg) / body weight (g) X± SEM
Normal	10	2.79 ±	0.38 3.80 ± 0.23
Group	9	1.02 ± 0. 32	4.01± 1.32
B Group	8	1.21 ± 0. 41	4. 213± 0.37
F Group	10	1. 18±0.46	4.45±1.63
G Group	8	1.28±0.2	4.47±1.24
H Group	8	1.34 ± 0. 43	4.67±0.48
I Group	7	1. 47 ± 0.28	4.56±0.62
K Group	9	1.43±0.36	4.89±1.47
CII Group	5	1.96±0.37	5.12 ± 1.56

Note: * indicates $P < 0.05$ compared with the control group:
* * means $P < 0.01$ compared with normal control group

Table 6

Comparison of wet weight of immune organs between cases with complete or significant regression of tumors in CII group and cases with no significant regression of other tumors in the same group

Immune organs (mg/g)	Normal group (N=10X±SEM)	Tumor regression group (N=10X±SEM)	Tumor non-regression group (N = 5X±SEM)
Thymus	2.79 ± 0.38	4. 65 ± 2.21**△△	1. 96 ± 0.37
Spleen	3.80 ± 0.23	10. 15 ± 2.29**△△	5. 12 ± 1.56

Note:

** indicates that the tumor is compared with the normal control group $P < 0.01$:
△△ indicates that the tumor regression group is compared with the tumor non-regression group $P < 0.01$.

6. Comparison of pathological results

In this experiment, pathological anatomy and pathological slice or section observation were performed on mice in each experimental group. Observed in detail the tumor infiltration, metastasis and changes in immune organs such as thymus and spleen; tumor tissue, lung, kidney, thymus, spleen and other organs were retained for histopathological section observation.

The results show that with the progression of the tumor, the local infiltration of the tumor expands and the tumor increases.

No obvious distant organ transfer was found.

Thymus atrophy is obvious and is positively correlated with tumor progression.

The spleen showed hyperemia and swelling.

In the recent observation group of triple cell transplantation, in cases where the tumor completely or significantly regressed, the thymus, spleen and liver were not significantly enlarged, and they also showed significant differences compared with the normal group. When the tumor completely subsided and the autopsy was performed, no residual cancer cells were found in the original tumor inoculation site under the naked eye and under the microscope.

At 3 and 4 weeks when tumor necrosis was most obvious, tumor tissue was collected for pathological section observation.

It was found that a large number of lymphocytes infiltrated around the tumor tissue and in the interstitial, formed a wrap around the tumor tissue, and the tumor cells were liquefied and coagulated and necrotic.

The pathological section of the immune organs showed thickening of the thymus cortical area, dense lymphocytes, increased epithelial reticulocytes, phagocytosis, and an increase in thymus bodies.

The white pulp area of the spleen is enlarged, the lymph nodules are increased, and the lymph cells are dense.

The tumor-bearing tumor tissue sections showed that the tumor cells infiltrated into the deep muscle tissue. There were tumor thrombi formed by tumor cell transplantation in the blood vessels, and there was no lymphocyte infiltration.

The thymic cortex is atrophy, the cells are sparse, the blood vessels are congested, and the lymphocytes in the spleen are significantly reduced and the cells are sparse. Tumor sections of other treatment groups showed clear borders around the cancer, with a small amount of lymphocyte infiltration around them, thymus and spleen changes between the triple group and the control, the cells were densely arranged and showed slight atrophy.

(3) Discussion

1. The efficacy evaluation

According to the above experimental results, adoptive immunotherapy of embryonic-derived immune cell transplantation can inhibit tumor growth to varying degrees, improve quality of life, mediate complete or partial tumor regression, significantly improve immune indicators, and prolong survival.

It shows that the transplantation of embryonic-derived immune cells does have the function of rebuilding tumor-bearing anti-tumor immunity.

Among them, it is best to carry out combined reconstruction of central and peripheral immunization at the same time, followed by partial reconstruction with dual and single cell transplantation.

2. The possible mechanism of action

The author believes that the possible mechanism of the action mainly has the following aspects:

① After the tumor-bearing body undergoes allogeneic embryonic cell transplantation, the body's immune system is **non-specifically stimulated**, and immune hyperplasia occurs to improve anti-tumor immune function.

② Cell transplantation belongs to the category of organ transplantation, and can continue to maintain vitality in the recipient for a certain period of time. **The tumor-bearing body receives embryonic-derived immune cell transplantation, and fetal liver cells provide multipotent thousand lymphocytes, combined with thymocyte and spleen cell transplantation.** And it is to achieve the joint reconstruction of intermediate immunity and peripheral immunity, so that the tumor-bearing body acquires adoptive immune function.

Numerous internal and external studies on the proliferation, differentiation, and function of embryonic immune organs, tissue cells, and embryonic immune organs showed a marked proliferation response to mitogens at 16W, and were significantly enhanced at 24W, which was significantly higher than adults.

At 8W of pregnancy, lymphoid tissue began to appear in the embryonic thymus, and at 20W, lymphoid masses and cells with secreted substances appeared.

The above studies all show that embryonic immune cells already have their own ability to exert immune responses in vivo.

③Some studies have shown that the supernatant and thymus extract of embryonic thymus tissue cultured in vitro can **significantly promote the E-garland formation rate and lymphocyte transformation of the receptor**. Through embryonic fetal immune cell transplantation, the cellular immune function of the tumor-bearing body can be improved.

④ *The low immunogenicity of the embryonic organs* and the **homology of the transplanted embryonic immune organs and the recipient's immune organs are conducive to the recipient's immune tolerance to the graft, and no transplant rejection (or mild rejection) occurs.** And they can stimulate each other to produce a synergistic effect to achieve the purpose of restoring and rebuilding immune function.

⑤ In addition, triple-cell transplantation-grade efficacy is superior to other treatment groups. The author believes that it is the result *of synergy due to the completion of a more complete central immune and peripheral immune simultaneous reconstruction.*

In short, its mechanism of action is far more than the above-mentioned simple, very complicated.

If it can detect the level of IL2, TNF, INF and other immune factors closely related to tumor immunity in peripheral blood, and the activity of immune cells directly related to tumor immunity such as NK, LAK, and TIL, and it is to mark or label the transplanted cells to find out their distribution and survival fate in the recipient, it will help to further clarify the mechanism of action.

3. About transplantation barrier

Although the embryonic organs have low immunogenicity, rejection is still inevitable, only the degree of severity, there is a problem of transplantation barrier.

It is directly related to the success or failure of transplantation and whether the graft can continue to function in the recipient.

The animals used in this experiment are all closed group hybrids, which to a large extent ensure that each experimental rat has a relatively close genetic background.

The animals used in this experiment are all closed-group hybrids, which to a large extent ensures that each experimental mouse has a relatively close genetic background.

In addition to the low immunogenic properties of embryonic tissue, this may be an important reason for successful transplantation without tissue matching.

In addition, it is also possible whether the cases with insignificant efficacy in the CI group and the CII group are caused by a mismatch in histocompatibility.

Therefore, studying and solving the problem of transplantation barrier may be the key to improving the efficacy.

4. **The selection of transplantation methods and methods**

The transplantation of embryonic immune organs from cell level, tissue level to whole organ level belongs to the category of adoptive immunity.

According to the current report, direct intra-blood cell transplantation of fetal liver and spleen cells is best, and thymus and spleen are best embedded in tissue omentum.

The cell transplantation technique is simple, easy to succeed but has a short maintenance time.

Therefore, the best transplantation path needs further observation and research.

Two

The progress and advances in research on tumor-inherited immunotherapy with embryonic-derived immune cell transplantation

A large number of clinical and experimental studies have confirmed that the immune function of tumor-bearing organisms shows a trend of progressive suppression as the course of the tumor progresses.

How to rebuild the anti-tumor immune function of the tumor-bearing body is the core content of tumor immunotherapy research?

Tumor Biotherapy Rising in the 1980s-----The fourth-generation oncology treatment program has brought oncology to a new era. One of the most prominent achievements is the adoptive immunotherapy of tumors.

The remarkable efficacy of LAK, TIL, and genetically modified TIL adoptive immunotherapy, represented by Roseoberg, for a variety of conventional treatment ineffective patients with advanced tumors has attracted worldwide attention.

This technology requires a large amount of high-purity artificially synthesized IL-2 obtained through bioengineering technology, and long-term in vitro culture and expansion to obtain a sufficient amount of immunologically active cells for reinfusion to achieve the goal, so the cost is expensive.

This research is still being carried out in depth.

A few domestic qualified units are also conducting research in this area.

This undoubtedly represents a very promising research direction in the field of cancer treatment, but it is still difficult to promote in China.

Embryo-derived immune cells, tissues and organ transplantation for tumor adoptive immunotherapy is another promising research content of tumor adoptive immunotherapy. It has the characteristics of simple technology, low cost and easy promotion.

In recent years, many domestic authors have used embryonic-derived liver, spleen, and thymus to study the transplantation of cells and tissues to organs with vascular pedicles for the treatment of advanced malignant elbow tumors. They have achieved certain results and gradually attracted people's attention.

(One)

Research Overview of Fetal Hepatocyte Transplantation (FLT)

In 1958, Uphoff first achieved a significant effect on promoting hematopoietic recovery after transfusion of fetal liver cells with lethal dose radiation. Since then, extensive research has been conducted on the use of fetal liver cell transplantation in patients with hematopoietic system diseases and malignant tumors after radiotherapy and hematopoietic suppression recovery after chemotherapy.

Subsequent research found that FLT not only has the function and role of rebuilding blood, but also has the role of rebuilding immune function. Research by Wu Zuze and others found that FLT has the function of reconstructing B lymphocytes.

They conducted a comparative study on the proliferation and differentiation characteristics of fetal hepatocytes and bone marrow hematopoietic stem cells, and found that fetal liver and spleen nodule-forming vascular cells possessed the basic characteristics of a variety of hematopoietic stem cells or lymphatic myeloid stem cells.

Fetal liver cells also contain a small amount of macrophages and lymphocytes. After 5 months of pregnancy, T lymphocyte content gradually increases.

It is believed that this is the material basis for FLT to treat certain hematopoietic disorders or immunodeficiency diseases with rebuilding blood function and immune function.

These characteristics of fetal hepatocytes, especially their immune rebuilding function, make FLT more important in improving the immune function of tumor patients. In recent years, there have been more and more research reports on the application of FLT in cancer treatment.

(Two)

The research on fetal spleen cell transplantation for tumor treatment

1. Research on the relationship between spleen and tumor growth.

Old et al. took the lead in studying the effect of the spleen on tumor growth, which has a history of 30 years.

During this period, many scholars have done a lot of experimental and clinical research on the role of the spleen in tumor immunity, and opinions have not yet reached a consensus.

It is believed that the spleen has positive and negative functions in tumor immunity.

With the in-depth study of splenic surgery and splenic function, most scholars tend to affirm the anti-tumor immune function of the spleen:

The spleen is the body's largest immune organ, where Th and Ts cells mature, and its secreted antibodies, immune factors such as Fibronetin, Tufftsinr-INF and IL-2, and tumor killer cells such as LAK and NK play important roles in tumor immunity.

Ge Yigong and others found that the effect of splenectomy on the growth of rat W256 sarcoma found that the survival rate of tumor inoculation and tumor diameter in the spleen-excision group were significantly higher than those in the control group. It showed a decrease in total T and Th cells, a slight increase in Ts cells, and continued low levels after tumor inoculation, which was very significantly different from the tumor-free and tumor-bearing control groups (P <0.001).

This is consistent with the results of our previous studies on the effect of spleen on tumor growth.

They also found that the decrease in the Th / Ts ratio of T cell subsets after spleen excision was positively correlated with tumor spread and metastasis. Lersch reported that lymphocytes in the spleen of tumor-bearing mice decreased progressively with tumor growth, consistent with our results.

The above research shows that the spleen plays an important role in tumor immunity.

2. Research on fetal spleen cell transplantation for tumor treatment

Based on the understanding of the role of the spleen in tumor immunity, many scholars have carried out clinical and experimental studies on fetal spleen cells and tissue transplantation for tumor treatment.

Ma Xuxian and others reported that 9 cases of various types of advanced malignant tumors treated with fetal spleen cell transplantation improved to varying degrees.

The author also observed in the study of the effect of the spleen on tumor growth that fetal spleen cell transplantation can significantly inhibit tumor growth. In addition, some authors also conducted a study on the characteristics and pathways of fetal spleen cell transplantation, and found that cell transplantation is best by intravenous route, followed by intramuscular and intraperitoneal injections, and tissue grafts are best for intraocular implantation. Both HVGR and GVHR Rare. The mechanism of splenocyte transplantation is still under study.

(Three)

Overview of research on embryo thymus transplantation for tumor treatment

The immune organs have the closest relationship with tumor immunity, and the most in-depth study is the thymus. The thymus is the central immune organ, where T cells develop and mature, and plays a decisive role in cellular immunity and even the entire immune regulation.

1. Study on the relationship between thymus and tumor growth

Thymus functional status is closely related to the occurrence of tumors. Tumors can lead to atrophy of the thymus, low levels of thymosin or similar thymic factor deficiency.

2. Application of embryo thymus transplantation in tumor treatment

Embryo thymus transplantation is used for tumor treatment, and many scholars have conducted extensive research.

Zhou Shifu and other 14 patients with tumors were treated with embryonic thoracic tissue transplantation. Immunity indicators improved after 46 hours, and the patient's condition was relieved and improved to varying degrees.

Song Ruzhe et al. Used fetal thymus tissue omentum meat transplantation to treat 10 cases of advanced malignant tumors, and achieved the same effect.

Liu Dungui and others respectively used cell transplantation, tissue transplantation and vascularized thymus transplantation to treat advanced liver cancer, and achieved a significant reduction in tumors in some cases and an average survival time of 6 months.

This shows that embryo thymus transplantation is an effective way for tumor immunotherapy. In addition, some authors have studied the activity of embryonic-derived immune organs at different gestational ages, retention time and other characteristics, and found that the fetal organs have better activity after 5 months of pregnancy. Studies on the transplantation route show that fetal liver cells and spleen cells are transplanted. Intravenous infusion is preferred, thymocytes are preferably injected intramuscularly, and spleen and thymus tissue transplantation is preferably embedded in the omentum. The above studies have provided valuable theoretical and experimental basis for adoptive immunotherapy of embryo-derived uterine transplantation for tumor adoptive immunotherapy, which will be helpful for future research.

10

The article V

**The inhibitory effect of Huang Lateng ethyl acetate
extract on tumor neovascularization in mice**

Since Folkman proposed or put forward the concept that tumor growth depends on blood vessel formation in 1971, the <u>successive studies have further confirmed that blood vessel growth is a key precondition or prerequisite for tumor development.</u>

As a result, people correspondingly proposed the concept of anti-angiogenesis therapy, which is to prevent the formation or establishment of small solid tumors by preventing the formation of new blood vessels and/or the expansion of the new blood vessel network and/or destroying the new blood vessels to prevent the growth, development and metastasis of tumors.

At present, foreign countries have done a lot of research in this aspect and made gratifying progress, which is expected that it will be used as an effective means of treating tumors. However, the domestic research on preventing tumor neovascularization started late and there are few reports. There are only some reports of counting the microvessel density of tumor tissue.

With the continuous in-depth research on Huang Lateng, its new pharmacological effects have also been discovered.

<u>For example, anti-tumor effect and two-way regulation of the immune system. In particular, the recently discovered Huang Lateng inhibits the migration, proliferation and differentiation of vascular endothelial cells to form a lumen in vitro, suggesting that it has a better inhibitory effect on angiogenesis.</u>

In order to further explore the inhibitory effect of Huang Lateng on tumor neovascularization in vivo, we adopted a mouse abdominal muscle transplanted tumor model, on the basis of observing the characteristics of tumor blood vessel formation and its relationship with tumors, according to the new research findings in recent years and our own experimental results----------Huang Lateng has a dose-dependent two-way regulation effect on the immune system, it is to choose the appropriate dose of Huang Lateng Acetate Acetate Extract (TG) that does not affect the immune function of the body to conduct experimental research on the inhibitory effect of tumor angiogenesis in mouse abdominal muscle transplantation, in order to understand the performance of TG in inhibiting tumor angiogenesis and to provide experimental reference for further anti-tumor research from the perspective of blood vessels.

One. Experimental Study on Observation of Neovascularization of Tumor Transplanted in Mouse Abdominal Muscle

Experimental study on observation of neovascularization of tumors transplanted in abdominal muscles of mice

In this experiment, according to the anatomical position and structural characteristics of the abdominal muscles of mice, the animal model with transplanted EAC tumor in the abdominal muscles was used, and the blood vessels were fixed and displayed by the method of transparent specimens in order to understand the characteristics of tumor blood vessels formation and its relationship with tumors.

[Experiment 1] [Experiment 1]
(1) Materials and methods (1) Materials and methods

1. Material

(1) Animals:

There are 20 Kunming mice weighing 18-22 g, half male and half female.

(2) Cancer bearing mice:

Kunming mice are intraperitoneally inoculated with EAC cells.

(3) Apparatus and instruments:

Mouse fixing plate, 1ml syringe, test tube and heparin tube, glass slide, ophthalmic surgical scissors, microsurgery scissors and surgical forceps, small triangular needle, 1-0 silk thread, ophthalmic needle holder, glass plate, optical microscope, BH-2 Olympus Japan-made microscopic observation and photography system.

(4) Reagents:

Wright's dye solution, 0.2% trypan blue saline solution, Hank's solution, hair removal agent, 1% sodium pentobarbital solution, 10% formaldehyde solution, 70%, 80%, 90%, 95% and 100% Butanol solution, wintergreen oil.

2. Method

(1) Preparation of EAC cell suspension (6.0×10^7/ml):

It is aseptically to extract the ascites of cancer-bearing mice that have been inoculated for 7-9 days into a sterile test tube, and take a small amount of it in heparin for cell counting, and store it around with ice cubes.

Place the remaining abdominal fluid water droplets in the needle with the hole on a glass slide, push the slide, Wright staining, and then perform cell classification and counting. Among them, the cancer cells should be >>95% (if insufficient, do not select mice).

Then take the ascites in the heparin tube and dilute it with normal saline 10 times and 100 times, take 0.95ml each plus 0.1ml of 0.2% trypan blue saline solution, mix it, and count the total number of tumor cells and dead tumor cells by white blood cell counting method.

Then take the ascites in the heparin tube and dilute it with normal saline 10 times and 100 times, then take 0.95 ml each plus 0.1 ml of 0.2% trypan blue saline solution, mix well, count the total number of tumor cells and dead tumor cells by white blood cell counting method, and calculate Its survival rate. It should be ≥95% (if not enough, do not select a rat).

Finally, the ascites in the test tube is diluted with sterile pre-chilled Han k's solution to a concentration of 6.0×10^7ml, which is used for inoculation.

(2) Vaccination or inoculation in the peritoneum:

After 2 days in advance, the mice whose abdominal hair was depilated with the depilatory agent were anesthetized by intraperitoneal injection of 1% pentobarbital (0.3 mg/10 g body weight). And then fixed on the mouse board in a supine position, disinfected the abdominal skin. Then it is to cut the skin about 1.2cm in length from the lower edge of the center of the xiphoid process about 1cm, or cut the skin about 1.2cm long from the center of about 1cm below the xiphoid process, and gently and meticulously separate it to one side. Look for areas with few blood vessels. Inoculate

0.04 ml of EAC cell suspension at a concentration of 6.0×10^7/ml into the abdominal muscles. It can present a relatively full little "piqiu" without collapsing. It means that the peritoneum has not been penetrated and the inoculation site is correct.

Finally, the skin is sutured and isolated and protected until the animal is safe and sober.

The note:

During the inoculation process, the test tube containing the cancer cell suspension should always be placed in ice to ensure that its survival rate remains unchanged, and the operation should be as fast and stable as possible.

(3) Production of grouping and transparent specimens:

The 20 inoculated mice were randomly divided into 10 groups according to 2 in each group.

Starting from the first day after the inoculation, a group of mice were sacrificed by cutting off the cervical vertebrae every day to make transparent specimens.

The specific production process is as follows:

The sacrificed mice were placed in a 10% formaldehyde solution and fixed for 24 hours.

Place the sacrificed mice in a 10% formaldehyde solution for 24 hours.

Take it out, cut the skin, peel off the entire abdominal muscle membrane, rinse with distilled water for 1 minute, and put in different concentrations of tert-butanol (70%, 80%, 90%, 95%. 100%) for dehydration for 6-8 hours. And finally put it directly into wintergreen oil until the tissue is completely transparent.

(4) Observe and photograph tumor blood vessels:

Observe the transparent specimen in a small plate filled with wintergreen oil with a BH-2 Olympus microscope, and pay attention to the shape, number and distribution of new microvessels around and in the tumor tissue. Then take a photomicrograph.

The Olympus microcirculation photomicrography system was used to observe the flow rate of new microvessels.

(5) The Results

On the first day after inoculation, no new blood vessels grew in the inoculated area, and there was slight oozing of the original host microvessels around it.

On the second day, the tumor cell mass increased. It was seen that the slender and curved new blood vessels from the original host microvessels entered the tumor.

The discontinuous blood vessel segments were also seen in the tumor.

On day 3-4, the tumor tissue further grows, the density of new blood vessels outside the tumor increases, the diameter of the tube is irregular, and the arrangement is disordered; there are obvious discontinuities, incomplete, uneven distribution, and different thicknesses in the direction of the muscle fibers in the tumor. Some of the new blood vessels are dotted or bud-shaped, and the blood vessels can be connected by irregular bud-shaped blood vessels.

On days 5-6, the tumor grows aggressively, and the microvessels outside the tumor are tortuous, dilated, or distributed in clusters with uneven thickness; the blood vessels inside the tumor begin to interweave or expand in a sinus shape.

On days 7-8, the tumor appeared red. The microvessels outside the tumor are dilated, tortuous and have various shapes; except for a few discontinuous short and small blood vessels scattered irregularly in the tumor, the morphology of the blood vessels is not clear, and most of them are fused into sheets or masses.

By day 9-10, only red zones fused into a mass were seen in the tumor, with brown hemorrhage and necrosis in the center, and extremely dilated and deformed blood vessels could be distinguished in some areas.

Through the mouse abdominal muscle transplantation tumor model, it can be more intuitively observed or it is possible to observe more intuitively from the "inflammation"-like changes that stimulate blood vessel growth on the first day after vaccination to the gradually formed tumor blood vessels in the future, which reflects the formation characteristics of tumor neovascularization and its relationship with tumors:

Tumor newly formed microvessels are generally characterized by curving, disorderly arrangement, irregular tube diameter, lack of continuity and integrity, and even appearing like comma or bud-like differentiation and immature differentiation.

It even has the characteristics of comma-like or bud-like differentiation naïve and immature.

The relationship between it and the tumor is manifested by the continuous proliferation and expansion of tumor cell clusters with the formation and growth of new microvessels in the inoculated area.

At the same time, the progressively growing tumor mass increases the pressure, **dilation, and necrosis of the central blood vessel, which is manifested as a fusion mass with red color-like changes.**

Experimental study on the effect of different doses of TG on the immune function of mice

In recent years, there have been reports that Huang Lateng has a dose-dependent two-way regulation of immune function. TG is the refined product after repeated separation and extraction of the crude drug Huang Lateng.

To further understand its effect on the immune system, in this experiment three different doses of TG were selected to preliminarily reflect the effect of TG on mouse peritoneal macrophages (Macrophoge, Mφ) phagocytic function and immune organs to reflect its effect on mouse immune function.

[Experiment 2]

The effect of TG on the Mφ phagocytosis of the abdominal cavity

(1) Materials and methods

1. Material

(1) Animals:

Kunming mice weighing 18-22 g, half male and half female, total 40 mice.

(2) Drugs and reagents:

1. TG suspension:

After grind the yellow lateng acetate extract tablets into powder and use 0.5% light methyl cellulose (Carboxythmethyl cellulose, CMC) to prepare three different concentrations of suspension, namely TG1 10 mg/10ml, TG2 10mg/20ml, TG3 40mg/10ml;

2. 0.5% CMC solution;

3. 2% chicken red blood cell (CRBC) suspension:

Aseptically collect 2ml of blood from the inferior wing vein of the chicken in a heparin tube, wash with normal saline three times and discard the supernatant and interface white blood cell layer after centrifugation. After the hematocrit is constant, use normal saline to make 2% (V/V) Red blood cell suspension:

4. Sterile calf serum;

5. 1: 1 Acetone---methanol solution;

6. 4% (V/V) Giemsa-phosphate buffer

(3) Apparatus and instruments:

Gavage needle, incubator, and the rest, see [Experiment 1].

2. Method

(1) Grouping:

Forty mice were randomly divided into TC1 group, TC2 group, TC3 group and control group according to 10 mice in each group.

(2) Gavage:

Each of the above groups of mice was given 0.2ml/10g body weight with corresponding concentration of TG suspension (the dosage is 20 mg/kg body weight in TC1 group, 40 mg/kg body weight in TC2 group, and 80 mg/kg body weight in TC3 group) and 0.5% CMC solution for 12 days.

(3) Induction and functional measurement of abdominal cavity Mφ:

On the 10th day of intragastric administration, 0.5ml of calf serum was injected into the abdominal cavity of each mouse aseptically.

On the 13th day, each mouse was intraperitoneally injected with 1ml of 2% CRBC suspension, 30 minutes later, the cervical spine was removed and sacrificed. The abdominal skin was cut in the middle, and 2ml of normal saline was injected into the abdominal cavity and the mouse body was rotated. Aspirate 1ml of peritoneal lotion, and evenly drop them on 2 slides, put them in an enamel box pad with wet paper cloth, transfer to 37°C thermostat and incubate for 30 minutes, rinse in normal saline, dry, 1: 1 Acetone: fix with methanol solution, stain with 4% Giemsa-phosphate buffer, rinse with distilled water, and dry. <u>Finally, count the Mφ (200 per piece) under the oil glass of the microscope, and calculate the percentage of phagocytosis by the following formula.</u>

<u>Devouring percentage = Mφ devouring CRBC/200 Mφ X 100%</u>

(4) Statistical processing:

The data are expressed as mean ± standard error (X ± SD), and use t test.

(2) Results

The measurement results of TG on the Mφ phagocytosis of the mouse abdominal cavity are shown in Table as the following:

Table The effect of TG on the phagocytic function of mouse abdominal cavity (X±SD)

Group	Dose (mg/kg)	Number of cases	Number of swallowed CRBC (%)
Control group	---	10	44. 83 ± 0.41
TG1	20	10	47. 20 ± 0.35
TG2	40	10	45. 72 ± 0.25
TG3	80	10	44. 40 ± 0.45.
Note: Compared with the control group, P<0.05			

It can be seen from the above Table that TG can significantly activate the phagocytic function of Mφ at a low dose of 20 mg/kg body weight ((P <0.05), while a medium dose of TC of 40 mg/kg has no significant effect on the phagocytic activity of Mφ (P> 0.05), when the high dose of 80 mg/kg, the body weight showed the effect of inhibiting Mφ phagocytosis (P<0.05).

The above results show that TG can affect the phagocytic function of the mouse abdominal cavity Mcp, and has obvious dose-dependent characteristics, that is, with the gradual increase of the TG dose, the phagocytic function of the mouse abdominal cavity Mφ can be stimulated, without obvious influence and Inhibit 3 different effects.

[Experiment 3]

The effect of TG on the immune organs of young mice

(1) Materials and methods

1. Material

(1) Animals:

Kunming mice aged 3 weeks, weighing 10-12g, half male and half female, totaling 40 mice.

(2) Drugs:

TG suspension and 0.5% CMC solution: the preparation is the same as before.

(3) Apparatus and instruments: analytical balance, see [Experiment 1] for the rest.

2. Method

(1) Grouping and gavage: see [Experiment 1].

(2) Weigh the thymus and spleen:

On the 13th day of the experiment, the young mice were sacrificed by cervical dislocation. The skin, liver, thoracic cavity and abdominal cavity were cut, the thymus and spleen were completely removed, dried on filter paper and weighed with an analytical balance.

(3) Statistical processing:

The data are expressed as mean ± SD (X±SD), and t test is used.

(2) Results

See Table as the following for the weighing results of thymus and spleen.

It can be seen from Table as the following. Different doses of TG have different effects on the immune organs of young mice. The effect of TG on the thymus of young mice can increase weight at a lower dose (20 mg/kg body weight) (P<0.05).

Although there was a tendency to reduce weight at the middle dose (40 mg/kg), there was no significant difference from the control group (P>0.05);

The high-dose (80 mg/kg) thymus was significantly atrophied compared with the control group ((P<0.01).

The effect of TG on the spleen of young mice only showed the effect of inhibiting its growth at high doses (P<005), and there was no significant effect on it at medium and low doses (P>0.05).

Table The effect of TG on the immune organs of mice (X±SD)

Group	Dose (mg/kg)	Number of cases	Thymus weight (mg/10g body weight)	Spleen weight (mg/10g) weight
Control group	--	10	26. 38 ± 1	70.43±0,76
101	20	10	30. 20 ± 0	72.65±0.83
102	40	10	23.48±0.88	69.88±0.56
103	80	10	21.12±0.76	68.44±0.42'
Note: Compared with the staring group, P<0. 05; **P< 0,01				

Through the effect of TG on the phagocytic function of mouse abdominal cavity Mcp and the weight of the immune organs of young mice, it preliminarily reflects that TG has a dose-dependent two-way regulation effect on the immune function of mice, that is, with the increase of dose, it can be enhanced and not obvious. Affect and suppress 3 different immune effects. **It is suggested that the scope of application of TG can be expanded by choosing different doses of TG to produce different effects on the immune system.**

Experimental study on the inhibitory effect of different doses of Huang Lateng ethyl acetate extract on tumor neovascularization of abdominal muscle transplantation in mice

[Experiment 4]

Observation of neovascularization of tumors transplanted in abdominal muscles of mice

Recent studies have found that Huang Lateng has the characteristics of inhibiting **the migration and proliferation of vascular endothelial cells,** thereby inhibiting angiogenesis.

In order to further explore its inhibitory effect on tumor neovascularization, this experiment selected an appropriate dose of TG (40 mg/kg body weight) that does not affect the immune function of mice on the basis of the previous experiment, through intravital observation of microcirculation microscope, the inhibitory effect of tumor neovascularization on abdominal muscle transplantation in mice was studied.

(1) Materials and methods

1. Material

(1) Animals: Kunming mice weighing 18-22g, half male and half female, total 40 mice.

(2) 6.0×10^7/mIEAC cell suspension; see [Experiment 1] for preparation

(3) 20mg/10mgTG suspension and 0.5% CMC solution;

See [Experiment 2] for preparation

(4) ***HH-1 type microcirculation detection system*** (microcirculation microscope, photomicrography system and display system, video cursor blood flow meter, etc.), the other required reagents and instruments are described in the previous experiment.

2. Method

(1) Inoculation: see [Experiment 1]

(2) Grouping:

The 40 tumor-bearing mice inoculated were randomly divided into a treatment group and a control group, each with 20 mice, and each group was randomly divided into 4 groups, set as 3 days, 6 days, 9 days, 12 days group, each day for 5 mice.

(3) Gavage:

From the first day after inoculation, the administration group and the control group were analyzed by **intragastric administration of 20 mg/ml TG suspension and 0.5% CMC solution at 0.2ml/10g body weight**.

(4) **Observation of neovascularization of tumor:**

On the 3ʳᵈ, 6ᵗʰ, 9ᵗʰ and 12ᵗʰ days, the mice in the corresponding groups (namely, the 3 day group, the 6 day group, the 9 day group, and the 12 day group) of the two groups were observed to observe the neovascularization of the tumor.

The specific methods and steps are as follows:

①After intraperitoneal injection of 1% pentobarbital (0.3 mg/log body weight) anesthetized before operation, carefully cut the skin from under the xiphoid process to the lower abdomen, and bluntly separate the skin from the side of the tumor to the midaxillary line, and then cut the abdominal muscles with the white thread. The operation should be **meticulous and light**. If a little blood oozes, a small gauze with warm saline can be used to stop the bleeding.

② Place the mouse on its side on the self-made observation platform, turn the abdominal muscle on the free skin side over, and fix the edge of the incision on the edge of the small window on the observation platform, so that the half of the abdominal muscle covers the entire small window, and the tumor mass Located in the middle of the small window.

③Put the mouse observation platform on the microscope stage in the incubator (refer to the method introduced by Tianniu and improve the preparation method), and drip Ringer's solution at 37°C on the turned abdominal muscles to moisten the abdominal muscles.

④Start the cold light source and adjust the focus to observe.

(5) Observation items:

Use the HH-1 type microcirculation detection system to observe the shape and number of new microvessels in and around the tumor, and take photomicrographs:

It is to measure the density of new microvessels entering and leaving the tumor and the average diameter and flow velocity of the small arteries and veins of the tumor, using vernier calipers to measure the largest diameter and transverse diameter of the tumor, and calculate its largest transverse section or the maximum cross section.

(6) Statistically process the above data:

It is expressed as mean ± standard error (X ±SD), and t test is performed.

(2) Results

1. The changes in the morphology and number of new microvessels in and around the tumor are shown in the following Table and Figure.

Table The effect of TG on the morphology and number of new microvessels in and around the tumor

Observation days	Control group	TG medication group
3rd day	1.Obviously running new blood vessels can be seen in the tumor: 2. There are curved microvessels in and out of the tumor. 3.The whole tumor is light red.	1.No curved new blood vessels entered or left the tumor, and the blood vessels around the tumor grew straight in the original direction: no obvious new blood vessels were seen in the tumor. 2.The whole tumor is milky white.
Day 6	Around the tumor, a large number of microvessels of uneven thickness were separated from the host's small blood vessels, and then moved into the tumor and formed a network of scattered nodular capillaries, making the entire tumor pink.	Thinner spiral blood vessels can be seen around the tumor: new blood vessels appear in the tumor, but there is no expansion or distortion. The entire tumor is light red.

Day 9	A large number of twisted and expanded microvessels appeared around the tumor; a large number of new blood vessels were seen running inside the tumor, intertwined to form bundles, spirals, and pointed cone or sac-shaped new blood vessel buds. The tumor tissue is fleshy red	There were tortuous new blood vessels around the tumor, but not many: the blood vessels inside the tumor increased and began to expand irregularly. The whole tumor is light red
Day 12	A large number of peritumoral blood vessels are shaped like beads, or are intertwined to make the arrangement disorder, or extend into the tumor to form masses; the blood vessels in the tumor are extremely dilated and touch each other to form a block or anal sinus, forming a large area at the center. The light-transmitting necrotic bleeding area makes the tumor appear brownish red.	There are more new blood vessels around the tumor, but they are slender, and there is no intertwining phenomenon; the blood vessels in the tumor expand and merge, but necrosis and hemorrhage are seen. The tumor is fleshy red.

2. The density of new microvessels entering and leaving the tumor (number of new microvessels around the tumor cell cluster/mm2) is shown in Table as the following:

Table The effect of TG on tumor microvessel density (root/mm2) (X±SD)

Group	Number of cases	3rd day	Day 6	Day 9	Day 12
Control group	5	340 ± 0.14	8.34 ± 1.05	11.26 ± 1.28	13.1 ± 0.90
TG group	5	1.84 ± 0. 12**	3. 64 ± 0. 64**	6. 58 ± 1.20*	9.90 ± 0.92
Note: Compared with the control group *P<0.01, **P<0.05;					

The above results showed that the tumor microvessel density of the TG group was significantly lower than that of the control group (P<0.05), indicating that TG has the effect of inhibiting tumor microangiogenesis. It is especially on the 3rd and 6th day of age, the performance was more prominent (P<0.05).

At the same time, it can be seen from Figure that the microangiogenesis rate of the control group was faster in the first 6 days, and then gradually slowed down; while the microangiogenesis rate of the TG group in the first 6 days was slower than that in the last 6 days, and was significantly smaller than the control group, which showed that TG significantly slowed down the rate of microangiogenesis in the first 6 days and inhibited its growth.

The rate of microangiogenesis in the last 6 major TG groups gradually increased, and it was equivalent to the control group when it was 10-12 years old, indicating that the effect of TG on inhibiting microangiogenesis in the second 6 days began to weaken. However, it can be seen from the below table that at the 12th day, the density of neovascularization in the TG group was still significantly lower than that in the control group, indicating that the combined effect of the drug at this time still showed inhibition of tumor microvessel growth.

3. *The average tube diameter and flow velocity of the tumor-supplied fine arteries and veins*

The results are shown in Table 1, 2,3,4

Table 1 The influence of TG on the diameter (μm) of donor arterioles (X±SD)

Group	Number of cases	3rd day	6th Day	9th Day	12th Day
Control group	5	15.0 ± 0.71	18.8 ± 1.07	20.8 ± 0.84	21.4 2 0.75
TG group	5	14.2 ± 0.97	9.0 ± 1.14	18.0 ± 0.71	19.2 ± 0.58

Table 2 The influence of TG on the diameter of tumor donor vein (μm) (X±SD)

Group	Number of cases	Day 3	Day 6	Day 9	Day 12
Control group	5	22.6 ± 0,68	24.0 ± 0.71	25.6 ± 0.51	26.8 ± 0.58
TG group	5	22.4 ± 0.93	23.2 ± 0.86	23.4 ± 0.75	19. 2 ± 0.68

Table 3 The influence of TG on the flow rate of the
tumor donor artery (mm/s) (X±SD)

Group	Number of cases	3rd day	6th day	9th Day	12th Day
Control group	5	0.42 ± 0.014	0.45 ± 0.022	0.39 ± 0.011	0.36 ± 0.015
TG group	5	0.43 ± 0.018	0.47 ± 0.013	0.42 ± 0.012	0.41 ± 0.013

Table 4 The effect of TG on the flow rate of the
tumor donor fine vein (mm/s_) (X±SD)

Group	Number of cases	3rd day	6th Day	9th Day	12th Day
Control group	5	0.35 ± 0.016	0.32 ± 0.014	0.28 ± 0.014	0.23 ± 0.016
TG group	5	0.34 ± 0.014	0.35 ± 0.013	0.32 ± 0.012	0.29 ± 0.015

Note: Compared with the control group *$P<0.05$,

It can be seen from the above table that the diameter of fine arteries and veins in the TG group on the 9th and 12th day was significantly smaller than that of the control group ($p<0.05$).

There was no significant difference between the two on the 3rd day and the 6th day (($P>0.05$).

On the 12th day, the fine arteriovenous flow velocity of the TG group was faster than that of the control group (($P<O.O5$),

There was no significant difference between the same on the 3rd, 6th and 9th days ($P>0.05$).

This shows that TG has an effect on the small blood vessels of Harajuku soil as the donor blood vessels. It is especially in the late stage, it can participate in affecting the blood supply to the tumor by reducing the tube diameter and speeding up the flow rate.

4. The largest cross section of the tumor

The results are shown in the below Table.

Table The effect of TG on tumor size (X±SD) Unit: mm2

Group	Number of cases	3rd day	6th Day	9th Day	12th Day
Control group	5	9.46±0.65	21.78±1.90	34.11±1.62	65.99 ± 2.21
TG group	5	4.91±0.76	14. 01±1. 27	27. 09 ± 2.16	62.64 ± 2.45

Note: Compared with the control group *P<0.05; *p<0.01

The above results indicate:

TG showed inhibition of tumor growth in the first 9 days (P<0.05), especially in the first 6 days, this effect was more obvious (P<0.05). By the 12th day, there was no significant difference between the tumors in the TG group and the control group (P> 0.05).

It is suggested that TG can significantly inhibit tumor growth in the early stage, and the effect is weakened in the middle and late stages, and there is no obvious inhibition until the late stage.

[Experiment 5]

The Measurement or Determination of plasma endothelin (ET) in mice with transplanted abdominal muscle tumors

ET is a class of biologically active peptides synthesized by endothelial cells with a wide range of biological effects. Recently, more and more studies have shown that it is closely related to the occurrence and development of tumors, and can participate in and promote the formation of blood vessels. To further understand the effects of tumor and ET and TG on ET of tumor mice, the following experiments were carried out.

(1) Materials and methods

1. Material

(1) Animals: Kunming mice weighing 18-22g, half male and half female, 60 mice in total.

(2) 6.0×10^7/ml EAC cell suspension, 20 mg/10ml TG suspension and 0.5% CMC solution: prepare each at the same time.

(3) Endothelin is put into immune kit.

(4) SN-682 type radioimmunoassay 7 counter.

The remaining required reagents and see the previous experiment.

2. Method

(1) Group according to the following table and gavage:

Table Grouping and gavage of experimental mice

Animal (mice)	Group	Gavage/intragastric administration (0.2ml/10g)
20 non-vaccinated	normal group ① 10	normal saline X 6d
	normal group ② 10	normal saline X 12d
40 inoculations	Control group ①10	0.5% CMC X 6d
see (experiment 1	control group ②10	0.5% CMCX 12d
for the method)		
	administration group①10	20 mg/10ml TGX6d
	administration group ②10	20 mg/10ml TG X 12d

(2) ET measurement:

After administering for 6 days, take blood 2ml/mouse from the orbit of the mice in the normal group ①, the administration group ① and the control group ①, and place them in a test tube containing 10% EDTA·Na230ul and aprotinin 40ul.

Shake gently, 40°C Centrifuge at 3000 y pm for 10 minutes to separate the plasma and store at -20°C for testing.

After 12 days of administration, the remaining group of mice were taken blood and plasma separated by the same method, and the specific radioimmunoassay was used together with the plasma to be tested, and the SN-682 radioimmunoassay y counter was used for measurement. The operation was strictly in accordance with the instructions of the immune kit get on.

(3) Statistical processing:

Data are expressed as mean±standard error (X±SD), and comparison between groups is performed by analysis of variance F test.

(2) Results

The measurement results of mouse plasma ET are shown in the following Table:

Table The effect of TG on plasma ET in mice with transplanted abdominal muscle tumors (X±SD)

Unit: pg/ml

Group	Number of cases	6 days	12 days
Normal	group 10	93.6 ±4.72	93.4 ± 4.83
Control group	10	126.4 ± 3.87**	132.8 ± 4.0**
Administration group	10	106.4±4,49**△△	114.6±5.41*△

Note: Compared with the normal group, *P <0.05, **P<0.01; compared with the control group △P <0.05, △△P<0.01

The results show:

The ET of the administration group and the control group were significantly higher than that of the normal group ((P<0.05), indicating that the tumor can increase the plasma ET of mice. The ET of the administration group was significantly lower than that of the control group, and was significantly (P<0.05) <0.01), indicating that TG has the effect of reducing the increase in ET plasma caused by tumors, and the effect is stronger in the early stage.

The results of observing tumor neovascularization in mouse abdominal muscle transplantation using the microcirculation detection system show that:

1) TG can inhibit the growth of new microvessels in and around the tumor;

2) TG ReduceS the density of new microvessels entering and leaving the tumor;

3) TG Inhibit tumor growth, and have a significant effect in the early stage. In the late stage, the diameter and flow rate of the fine arteries and veins for the tumor are changed to reduce the diameter and increase the flow rate.

4) The measurement results of plasma ET show that tumors can increase plasma ET in mice, and TG has the effect of reducing the increase in plasma ET caused by tumors, and has a stronger effect in the early stage.

(3) Discussion

1. *Analysis on the establishment of a mouse abdominal muscle transplantation tumor model for the observation of neovascularization*

The methodology for evaluating and studying tumor microvessels is still in the stage of continuous exploration and improvement.

Most of the methods used in vivo **are rabbit cornea**, *chick embryo choriourea sac (CAM) and yolk sac, hamster cheek sac, rabbit ear chamber with artificial device and rat back subcutaneous air sac, also called "sandwich" observation room* as the transplanted tumor site to observe in vivo, or which is used as a site for tumor transplantion to observe in vivo.

In recent years, methods such *as corrosion casting and immunohistochemistry* have been used to display and identify vascular components.

The above methods have their own advantages and disadvantages. Recently, people are still exploring to find a simple, economical, quantitative, and highly repeatable model and method for studying angiogenesis.

For this reason, we combined the specific situation of our laboratory to study and design a mouse abdominal muscle transplantation tumor model, and improved the observation method of microcirculation to observe tumor neovascularization, which is simple, convenient and intuitive. Thus it has found a new way to study tumor microvessels in methodology.

(1) Model evaluation

Using tumor transplantation on mouse abdominal muscles to study and observe the relationship between tumors and blood vessels and the effects of drugs on tumor blood vessels has a reliable theoretical and practical basis.

The abdominal muscle layer of mice is thin, with a thin layer of fascia between the outer skin and the skin, and the inner and peritoneum are closely connected.

The blood circulation is provided by the arteries and veins under the abdominal wall and the arteries and veins under the abdominal wall.

Each branch is divided into small branches (arterioles and veins) and capillary branches, and a richer anastomosis is formed around the abdominal muscles on each side.

There are few vascular branches and anastomoses in the middle part, forming a sparsely vascularized area, which is convenient for observing new microvessels in this area.

When the EAC cell suspension is injected into the abdominal muscle layer, the tumor cells grow infiltratingly in the muscle layer and expand along the plane of the abdominal muscles, but do not adhere to the skin and abdominal viscera or organs.

When the tumor grows to a certain extent, it gradually breaks through the muscle layer, easily penetrates the peritoneum inward, and transfers to various organs in the abdominal cavity through implantation and produces ascites.

Therefore, it is better to choose to inoculate in the sparsely vascularized area, and to observe the tumor microvessels before the tumor has penetrated the peritoneum. It is not only convenient to observe the occurrence and changes of the neovascularization of the tumor on the side, but also to avoid the retroperitoneal penetration.

It can also avoid the compound influence of various factors on tumor neovascularization caused by ascites and tumor spread after penetrating the peritoneum.

In combination with the contents of this experiment, in order to better reflect and observe the whole process of the development of the tumor and its new microvessels transplanted in the abdominal muscles after repeated experiments, finally, a 6.0x10ml concentration of EAC cell suspension was selected for inoculation.

According to the growth status of the tumor, 10 days as the total number of observation days, 12 days as the total number of days for treatment.

The 3rd, 6th, 9th, and 12th days are used as the division points of the time period to reflect the response of the tumor to the drug in the early, middle and late stages of growth.

Mouse abdominal muscle transplantation tumor models can more intuitively and clearly reflect the formation and changes of tumor neovascularization, which provides new ideas and new methods for the study of tumor neovascularization in the selection of transplantation sites and the preparation of animal models.

The following points should be noted when preparing this model:

① The inoculation site should be selected in the abdominal muscles in the area with few blood vessels, and cannot penetrate the peritoneum. The sign is that there is a relatively full small "skin hill" at the inoculation site and does not collapse.

② The experimental operation should be gentle and meticulous, try to avoid the small vein branches (usually only 1-2) from the skin and the abdominal muscles to avoid local hemorrhage, affecting the effect of inoculation and the growth of tumor neovascularization after inoculation.

③ Appropriately increase the number of experimental animals to reduce the error caused by the lack of blood vessels on the abdominal muscles of each mouse due to individual differences that may not be completely the same.

(2) The evaluation of observation methods

The observation of transparent specimens:

The mouse abdominal muscle------membrane tissue is thin, and after the transparent treatment, except for the blood vessel part which is red, the other parts are transparent.

The blood vessels can be clearly seen by the naked eye, and the morphology, distribution and interrelation of capillaries can be observed under a microscope, which is not only convenient and intuitive, but also retains the original appearance and sense of the whole blood vessel.

When making transparent specimens, no ink or other pigments are used for perfusion, and blood vessels are directly displayed through the natural color of the blood, which avoids the influence of the particle size, dispersion, and viscosity of the perfusate on the quality of the specimen after perfusion and improper perfusion pressure. The factor of morphological change makes the transparent specimen completely reflect the state of the living body, so that the displayed blood vessel is closer to the real.

Using a transparent specimen of the abdominal muscle membrane, various blood vessels on the abdominal muscles can be clearly displayed, including the peritumoral and intratumoral microvessels, morphology, distribution and local hyperemia, oozing, bleeding, etc,making it more convenient to observe the new capillaries inside and outside the tumor. But it can only observe the morphological changes of microvessels after death, and cannot reflect the state of blood flow.

Therefore, if combined with the observation of living blood flow and functional indicators, it will be more conducive to comprehensively understand the characteristics of tumor neovascularization.

The Microcirculation microscope in vivo observation:

The mouse abdominal muscle---membrane is thin and membrane-like, it is easy to transmit light, and its blood vessel shape and flow state can be clearly seen through a microscope.

When the tumor cells are inoculated, they expand and grow in the abdominal muscles.

In the early stage, due to the insignificant increase in thickness, light can still be transmitted and the vascular morphology in the tumor tissue can be observed.

In the late stage, the tumor tissue grows and thickens, the central pressure increases, necrosis and hemorrhage appear, and it appears as an opaque solid mass. The blood vessels in this part can be seen clearly, but the blood vessels in other light-transmissive parts in the tumor can be seen.

Observation of new microvessels inside, outside and in and out of the tumor transplanted in mouse abdominal muscles and small arteries and veins through the microcirculation microscope can comprehensively reflect the relationship between tumor and blood vessels and the effect of drugs on tumor microvessels from the vascular morphology and flow pattern Impact.

The combination of the above two observation methods can complement each other. Observation of transparent specimens makes up for the inability to observe the blood vessels in the opaque area of the tumor in vivo, while in vivo observation supplements the inability to observe blood flow dynamics in transparent specimens. Because the above methods can only be used for one-time observation and cannot be used for long-term continuous dynamic monitoring, they also have shortcomings.

In order to be more accurate and in-depth research, further improvement and perfection of methodology are needed.

2. *Evaluation of experimental drugs*

Huang Lateng refers to the genus Euonymus Huang Lateng. There are 3 species in my country, namely Huang Lateng, Kunming Mountain crabapple and Northeast Huang Lateng (also known as black vine).

Its taste is pungent and bitter. It has the medicinal properties of "cold" and "heat".

(1) Evaluation of experimental drugs

Huang Lateng refers to the genus Euonymus Huang Lateng. There are three species in my country, namely **Huang Lateng**, **Kunming Mountain crabapple** and **Northeast Huang Lateng** (also known as black vine).

It tastes pungent and bitter, and has the medicinal properties of "cold" and "heat".

It can enter the liver and spleen meridian, pass 12 meridians, *clear heat and detoxify, dispel wind and remove dampness, relax muscles and activate blood, relieve swelling, relieve pain,* and *kill insects, anti-itch and other effects*

It was first collected in "Shen Nong's Materia Medica" and contains about 70 ingredients.

Since its use in the treatment **of rheumatoid arthritis** achieving certain curative effects in the 1970s, it has been widely used in the treatment of *chronic nephritis, hepatitis, thrombocytopenic purpura and various skin diseases* in the past 20 years.

At the same time, the research on its pharmacological effects has become more and more in-depth, covering a wide range of adrenal glands, immunity, reproduction, urine production, central nervous system and blood system, etc., and it is agreed that it can enhance ***adrenal cortex function, anti-inflammatory and analgesic, anti-fertility and anti-tumor activity.***

However, reports on its impact on the immune system are inconsistent, and there have been many disputes or controversies and reasoning which have occurred.

In the early days, people began to study the immune system because of its unique effects in the treatment of rheumatoid diseases.

The initial results showed that it suppressed immunity. With more and more in-depth research, most researchers gradually tended to the "two-way regulation" view, that is, the effect of Huang Lateng on immune function has a dose-dependent two-way regulation.

For example, Zheng Jiarun, Yan Biyu, Luo Dan, Lei Zhuo, Fan Yongyi, etc. respectively reported on the weight of mouse thymus, human thymocyte proliferation, mouse spleen cell NK activity, mouse spleen T cell and B cell function, T cell in vitro Proliferation has a two-way regulatory effect.

We tested the effects of different doses of TG on the function of mouse abdominal Mφ and immune organs, which also reflected the two-way regulation of Huang Lateng on the immune system.

The above results indicate that Huang Lateng is not only immunosuppressive.

Many experiments have confirmed that it often exhibits a certain degree of immune enhancement response at small doses, and within a certain dose range, it can appear reversible performance of enhancement and suppression, and it can show that it has almost no obvious impact on immune function.

The dose shows the effect of completely suppressing immunity. It significantly related to dose.

Based on the above conclusions, we choose the dose of TG that has no significant effect on the immune function for the experiment, which can avoid complicating the study of TG's inhibitory effect on tumor microvessels due to the influence of the drug on the immune function. At the same time, it also provides ideas and experimental exploration basis for further experiments and clinical studies of its anti-tumor effects on the premise that Huang Lateng does not damage the body's immune system.

Although the drugs selected in this experimental study are refined products after repeated separation and extraction, they contain a higher amount of active ingredients and have less side effects.

However, in order to further explore the effective components of the drug for suppressing blood vessels, it is still necessary to carry out the study of the chemical components and monomers after re-isolation and purification.

3. *Tumor angiogenesis characteristics*

Under normal circumstances, blood vessel formation is limited to embryonic development, wound repair, and endometrial regeneration, and the host can tightly control its birth through various mechanisms.

However, in tumors, people have not found any such mechanism to limit angiogenesis through research in the past 20 years, indicating that the formation of tumor blood vessels has its own characteristics.

Through the observation of new microvessels of transplanted tumors in the abdominal muscles of mice, we found that with the formation and growth of microvessels in this area, the tumor cell clusters continue to proliferate and expand in size, and the volume continues to expand.

The early manifestations are the exudation of the original host's microvessels, and the gradual beginning of slender and curved new microvessels, which are disorderly arranged, unevenly distributed, and irregular lumens, especially when the microvessels entering the tumor are discontinuous, lacking in integrity,

and some are present. The dots or buds indicate that it is immature and cannot form a complete and continuous basement membrane. It also lacks the sealing and wrapping of the differentiated multilayer structure of the blood vessel wall, which makes the blood vessel expand or appear as the nodular or sinus regular expansion

As the tumor grows progressively, a dark brown hemorrhage and necrosis area appears in the center. The blood vessels in the adjacent area are not easy to distinguish due to extreme expansion, which may be caused by the continuous proliferation of tumor cells leading to increasing intratumoral pressure.

Because the central part of the tumor has the highest pressure and is far from the new capillaries growing in from the outside of the tumor, necrosis in the central part is most likely to be found due to ischemia, including blood vessel necrosis and hemorrhage or bleeding.

However, there are always tumor microvessels with different shapes and active proliferation at the edge of the tumor to ensure the nutrient supply for its further invasive growth.

This phenomenon also illustrates the uncontrollability of its unlimited growth.

At present, people have adopted various methods to study tumor blood vessels.

The existing results have confirmed that the formation of tumor blood vessels is different from the formation of blood vessels under normal physiological conditions.

It has its own unique characteristics, such as naive differentiation, incomplete blood vessel walls, and no control by the body.

However, the whole process and regulation mechanism of its formation are still unclear, and it is still under exploration.

This experiment also only superficially reflects the relationship between tumor and blood vessels and some characteristics of tumor blood vessels.

If it is further studied, it needs to obtain a breakthrough in methodology, and from the **physiology and pathology** of blood vessel formation, **biochemistry, molecular biology** to continue to clarify the biological characteristics of its formation. In another word, for more in-depth research, it is necessary to obtain a breakthrough in *methodology*, **and continue to clarify the characteristics of its formation biology from the aspects of** *physiology and pathology* **of blood vessel formation,** *biochemistry, and molecular biology*.

4. The discussion on the inhibitory effect of TG on tumor neovascularization

Since Huang Lateng was discovered and applied, it has aroused widespread interest and attention in the medical circles at home and abroad, and has carried out or conducted multidisciplinary research and exploration on it in order to broaden its application range.

Recent studies have found that Huang Lateng has the characteristics of inhibiting *the migration and proliferation of vascular endothelial cells* (EC).

Zhu Jinbo and two Japanese scholars used the self-established EC strains F-2 and F-2 C to study the effect of Huang Lateng on the angiogenesis process. *The results show that Huang Lateng can directly act on EC, inhibit its migration, proliferation and differentiation, and form a lumen, suggesting that Huang Lateng has a better inhibitory effect on angiogenesis.*

We conducted experimental research on the inhibitory effect of Acetate Acetate Extract (TG) of Huang Lateng on the neovascularization of tumors transplanted into abdominal muscles in mice, and found that TG can inhibit tumor angiogenesis and has a significant early effect. Or it is speculated that its mechanism of action may have the following aspects:

(1) *Directly act on tumor neovascularization:*

It can be seen from the experimental results that TG can significantly inhibit the growth of new microvessels in and around the tumor, and reduce the density of new microvessels entering and leaving the tumor. *It is speculated that TG may directly act on tumor vascular endothelial cells, inhibit their migration and proliferation, and slow down the formation, differentiation and growth of tumor blood vessels.*

(2) Directly act on tumor cells:

The direct killing effect of TG on tumor cells is a result of early confirmation.

It is generally believed that it exerts its cytotoxic effect by directly interfering with tumor cell DNA replication and inhibiting the synthesis of RNA and protein.

In angiogenesis, tumor cells themselves can produce a variety of angiogenic factors, such as *fibroblast growth factor (FGF), angiogenesis, transfer growth factor (TG F), tumor necrosis factor (INF-2), etc*., and also certain chemical mediators can be released to induce blood vessel formation in the host and tumor.

All of the above substances released by tumor cells that can induce blood vessel formation are collectively referred to by Folkman as **"tumor angiogenesis factor"** (tumor angiogenesis factor, TAF). **TG can directly kill tumor cells to reduce the production of TAF, thereby indirectly inhibiting angiogenesis.**

(3) **Change tumor blood flow:**

The results of the measurement of the average diameter and flow velocity of the fine arteries and veins of the host tumor reveal that TG can change the blood flow in the tumor by **affecting the blood supply of the tumor, and affect the growth and changes of the tumor and its new microvessels.**

(4) Reduce plasma ET content:

Recent studies have shown that *ET has the following function:*

a. *it has the effect of a growth factor that promotes cell proliferation,*
b. *it can promote the growth of endothelial cells and the proliferation of vascular smooth muscle cells,*
c. *it is closely related to tumors.*
d. *It can promote the transcription and expression of proto-oncogenes,*
e. *and the growth and differentiation of tumors.*
f. *it can Increase the blood flow of tumor tissue and promote blood vessel formation.*

The measurement result of plasma ET in mice showed that the tumor was significantly higher than the normal group, which proved that ET is closely related to tumors, and tumors can increase plasma ET in mice.

The TG group was significantly lower than the tumor control group, indicating that TG can significantly reduce the high plasma ET content of tumor mice, and also reduce the tumor-promoting and angiogenic effects caused by ET.

In addition, in this experiment, the characteristic that TG inhibits tumor angiogenesis in the late stage is weaker than that in the early stage.

In addition to the pharmacological characteristics of TG itself inhibiting angiogenesis, it may also be related to the accumulation of drugs.

It is speculated that with the extension of the medication time, TG accumulates in the body and exerts its extensive pharmacological effects, thereby affecting its effect of inhibiting tumor angiogenesis.

The results of this study suggest that TG can inhibit tumor growth by inhibiting tumor microangiogenesis without significant effect on the immune system, and has a significant early effect, which provides a reference for further research on TG in multiple fields and perspectives *It also provides new ideas for the study of TG anti-tumor mechanism*.

Of course, this conclusion still needs to be verified by repeated experiments, and further in-depth research is needed through drug purification and methodological improvement.

Inhibiting the formation of new microvessels in tumors can inhibit tumor growth is a new view in oncology in recent years.

This topic or subject is based on the study of the formation characteristics of neovascularization of tumors transplanted in the abdominal muscles of mice and its relationship with tumors, and the dose-dependent two-way regulation effect of the acetyl acetate extract (TG) of Huanglateng on the immune system of mice, by selecting the TG dose (40 mg/kg body weight) that has no significant effect on the immune function of mice, it is to perform experiments on the influence of the *shape and number* of new microvessels in the tumor transplanted into the abdominal muscles of mice, *the density* of new microvessels entering and leaving the tumor, *the average diameter and flow velocity o*f the tumor donor arteries and veins, *tumor size and plasma ET*.

It was found that TG may directly act on tumor neovascularization and tumor cells, change tumor blood volume, reduce plasma ET content and other mechanisms to jointly exert the effect of inhibiting tumor angiogenesis, and the effect is significant in the early stage

The results of this study suggest that the study of TG's anti-tumor effect from the perspective of blood vessels is of certain significance, and it needs further research to confirm and in-depth.

Fourth, the significance of inhibiting tumor angiogenesis in treatment

Tumor formation is a complex process and is affected by many factors, including the establishment of tumor vascular network.

Many studies have proved that tumor growth must depend on angiogenesis.

By inhibiting certain steps or the entire process of tumor angiogenesis, the control of tumor growth is of great significance for tumor treatment and prevention of tumor metastasis.

1) *The relationship between tumor angiogenesis and tumor occurrence and growth*

At present, the research on how tumors occur is mainly focused on the study of oncogenes.

However, for the malignant transformation of tissues or the formation of a tumor, *the activity of oncogenes is only a necessary condition, not all.*

Folkman Judah of Harvard Children's Hospital studied *the occurrence of ß-cell tumors in the pancreatic islets of mutant mice,* which it was found that *the activity of oncogenes is related to the proliferation of ß-cells and during the occurrence of ß-cell tumors, angiogenesis plays an important role.*

The occurrence of tumor is due to the acquisition of the angiogenic ability of the hyperplastic tissue. The studies have confirmed that one of the obvious characteristics of most precancerous lesions is the lack of obvious neovascularization.

Compared with tumors with abundant angiogenesis, this point indicates that the progression of precancerous lesions to the vascular stage may be the "switch" of tumorigenesis.

This means that the induction of blood vessel formation and the subsequent formation of new blood vessels precede the formation of tumors.

Once a tumor is discovered, its further growth must rely on the continuous formation of blood vessels.

This concept was proposed by Folkman as early as 1971, and he believed that *tumor cells and blood vessels constitute a highly integrated ecosystem. Without angiogenesis, tumors cannot grow*.

In recent years, many experimental research evidences have further supported the above view.

The growth phase of solid tumor cells can be divided into *the avascular pre-invasive phase and the vascularized aggressive growth phase.*

In the early stage of invasion, the growth of tumor cells mainly depends on diffusion to obtain nutrition.

When the diameter of solid tumor exceeds 1-3 cm and the number of cells reaches about 10^7, blood vessels must provide oxygen and nutrients for its central part and continued growth.

1. **Observe the mouse melanoma cell group cultured in agar.**

When it grows to $1mm^3$, the proliferation of its peripheral cells is equivalent to the necrosis of the central cell.

The tumor continues to grow, and the proliferation and necrosis reach a dynamic balance.

If the tumor is growing in the body, it is also called the vascular stage of tumor growth.

If the tumor is growing in the body, it is also called the vascular stage of tumor growth.

Breaking this state requires new and functional capillary growth to provide sufficient oxygen and nutrient supply.

b. Observe the growth rate of the transplanted tumor in the hyaline cavity of the mouse. Before angiogenesis, the tumor grows linearly and slowly. After angiogenesis, the tumor grows exponentially and rapidly.

2. **Observe the growth rate of the transplanted tumor in the hyaline cavity of the mouse.**

Before angiogenesis, tumors grow linearly and slowly. After angiogenesis, tumors grow exponentially quickly

3. *The tumor tissue mass is implanted on the rabbit cornea.*

The tumor is at a distance from the host vascular bed.

It was found that the new capillaries grew from around the cornea to the tumor, with an average growth rate of 0.2 mm/d.

When the new blood vessels grow into the tumor, the tumor mass begins to grow rapidly and exceeds 1 cm^3.

4. **Growing tumors in isolated mouse perfused organs.**

Since there is no vascular proliferation, the tumor is limited to 1mm^3.

If transplanted to mice, the tumor rapidly grows to 1-2 cm^3 after angiogenesis.

e. Suspend tumor cells in the anterior aqueous humor of the eye. Because there is no blood vessel, the tumor growth is less than 1 m3. If the tumor is transplanted to the blood vessel of the iris, the tumor grows rapidly, reaching 1.6 times the original volume within 2 weeks.

5. Suspend tumor cells in the anterior aqueous humor of the eye,

Because there are no blood vessels, the tumor grows less than 1 mm³.

If the tumor is transplanted to the blood vessel of the iris, the tumor grows rapidly, reaching 1.6 times its original volume within 2 weeks.

6. Human retinoblastoma has metastasized to the vitreous or anterior chamber, and the growth of the tumor is restricted due to lack of blood vessels.

7. **Use 3H thymine to label and fix the cancer cells.**

The labeling index of tumor cells decreases as the distance from the nearest open capillary increases.

The average tumor cell marker index is a function of the tumor vascular endothelial cell marker index.

8. *Transplanted tumors in the chicken embryo chorionic sac (CAM).*

In the avascular period (> 72h), tumor growth is restricted. A set of experiments reported that the tumor diameter does not exceed 0.93±0.29 mm.

Within 24 hours after blood vessel formation, the tumor began to grow rapidly, and the average tumor diameter was 8.0±2.5mm on the 7th day.

9. Ovarian cancer that has metastasized to the peritoneum, before angiogenesis, it grows slowly, rarely exceeding 1 mm³.

10. It is found in rabbit membrane metastatic carcinoma that there is no angiogenesis in tumors with a diameter less than 1mm, while tumors with a diameter larger than it have angiogenesis.

All of the above indirectly or directly prove that tumor growth must depend on angiogenesis, and angiogenesis is a key prerequisite factor for tumor development.

2) **Anti-tumor effects of angiogenesis inhibitors**

In the early 1970s, as the concept of tumor growth relied on angiogenesis was put forward and researched, the concept of anti-angiogenesis treatment was also proposed correspondingly, or put forward accordingly, that is, by preventing the occurrence of new blood vessels and (or) the expansion and (or) destroy new blood vessels to prevent the generation or establishment of small solid tumors and prevent tumor growth, development and metastasis.

The ways to use anti-angiogenesis therapy are:

①*Inhibit tumor release tumor angiogenic factor (TAF)*

②*Neutralize the released TAF*

③*Inhibit the response of vascular endothelial cells (EC) to angiogenic factors*

④*Interference with the synthesis of basement membrane*

⑤ *Damage to new blood vessels formed by tumors, etc.*

In short, an ideal tumor angiogenesis inhibitor must be able to inhibit one or more steps of tumor angiogenesis, or the entire process.

At present, people have done a lot of research work in this area, and experimental results show that angiogenesis inhibitors (AI) can inhibit tumor growth, for example:

1) *Heparin plus hydrocortisone, which is widely reported in China, is recognized as an effective angiogenesis inhibitor.*

The experiments have confirmed that

1. *The combination of the two can inhibit the angiogenesis on the chick embryo chorioallantoic membrane (CAM), and can make tumor regression and prevent metastasis.*

2. It can also **inhibit rabbit corneal angiogenesis** caused by tumors.

3. When it is used to treat some mouse tumors, the effect is remarkable, in another word, it has significant effects when used to treat some mouse tumors, such as oral hepatic cord (200u/ml) and subcutaneous injection of cortisone (250mg), *100% reticulocyte sarcoma, 100% Lewis lung cancer and 80% B16 melanoma can be completely resolved. And 80% of tumors did not recur after regression.*

It can inhibit the proliferation of endothelial cells during in vitro experiments, inhibit tumor-induced angiogenesis during in vivo experiments, and inhibit tumor growth in mice. For example, 30 mg/kg can inhibit the growth of Lewis lung cancer and B16 melanoma.

2) *Fumagillin is an antibiotic naturally secreted by aspergillin.*

    a. In vitro experiments it can inhibit the proliferation of endothelial cells.

    b. In vivo experiments it can inhibit tumor-induced angiogenesis,

    c. And it can also inhibit tumor growth in mice, for example, 30 mg/kg can inhibit the growth of *Lewis lung cancer and B16 melanoma*.

3) **TNP-470** (*a synthetic analogue of fumagillin*) lug/ml can inhibit the growth of cultured *human umbilical vein endothelial* cells, 3-10 mg/kg can inhibit the *growth of human ovarian cancer transplanted* tumors in nude mice

4) **Platelet factor 4 (PF₄)** is a 28kd protein released from small particles when platelets aggregate or during platelet aggregation, and has a high affinity for heparin.

    a. Taytor et al. found that PF4 can newly inhibit the growth of CAM blood vessels.

    b. Recently, Maione et al. found that recombinant human PF4 (rHuPF4) can inhibit the proliferation and migration <u>of human endothelial cells and produce avascular areas in the CAM of chicken embryos</u>.

    c. Sharpe has confirmed that rHu PF4 has an inhibitory effect on the growth of solid tumors through studies on mouse melanoma and human colon cancer, in another word, Sharpe's studies on mouse *melanoma and human colon cancer* confirmed that rHu PF4 has an inhibitory effect on the growth of solid tumors.

5) *a-Difluoromethylornithine (DEMO)* is an irreversible inhibitor of ornithine destrengthase or deenzyme, which can inhibit the angiogenesis caused by melanoma on the CAM of chicken embryos, *thereby inhibited tumor growth on CAM.*

6) *Angiostain, a newly identified vascular inhibitor, is a 38kd protein that can inhibit endothelial cell production and angiogenesis in Lewis mouse tumors.*

When Folkman applied it to mice with metastases, the new inhibitor kept the metastases in a dormant state - the rate of tumor proliferation was equal to the rate of cell death.

In addition, it can also inhibit the growth of human tumors.

At present, people have realized that many anti-tumor methods, their anti-cancer effects directly or indirectly act on the structure or function of tumor blood vessels, such as anti-tumor angiogenesis, change of tumor blood flow and its regulation.

It is a new way to fight cancer by inhibiting the angiogenesis of malignant tumors to inhibit its growth and metastasis. At the same time, the use of angiogenesis inhibitors to treat tumors will start a new and promising field of clinical treatment, such as cooperation with surgery and chemotherapy, radiotherapy, immunotherapy, etc. will definitely improve the overall treatment level of tumors.

Tumor cells produce a variety of tumor angiogenesis factors (Tumor Angiogenesis Factor, TAF), such as basic fibroblast growth factor (b FGF),

Acidic Fibroblast Growth Factor (a FGF), Endothelial cell growth factor (ECGF), Vascular Endothelial Growth Factor (vEGF), Platelet Proendothelial Cell Growth Factor (PDECGF), Epidermal Growth Factor (EGF), Transforming growth factor (TG F, TGF B), Tumor Necrosis Factor (TGF), Granulocyte Colony Stimulating Factor (G-CSF),Granulocyte Macrophage Colony Stimulating Flash (GM-CSF) etc.

TAF plays a role in promoting tumor occurrence, development and metastasis.

It is one of the effective measures to prevent and treat tumors to explore the mechanism *of tumor microangiogenesis and inhibit the formation and growth of microvessels, or by exploring the mechanism of tumor microangiogenesis and inhibiting the formation and growth of microvessels.*

It may become a promising new anti-cancer therapy following surgery, radiotherapy, chemotherapy and biological therapy.

The series of Anti-cancer, anti-cancer metastasis research, scientific and technological innovation scientific and technological achievement

Part VI

The case list & some typical cases of XZ-C immune regulation and control anti-cancer Chinese medicine treatment of cancer

Part I

List of some cases of XZ-C immunoregulatory anti-cancer Chinese medicine for treatment of malignant tumors (with demograph information)

1. List of some cases of liver cancer treated by XZ-C immunoregulatory anti-cancer Chinese medicine

2. List of some cases of pancreatic cancer treated by XZ-C immunoregulatory anti-cancer Chinese medicine

3. List of some cases of gastric cancer treated by XZ-C immunoregulatory anti-cancer Chinese medicine

4. List of some cases of XZ-C immunoregulatory anti-cancer Chinese medicine for treatment of lung cancer

5. List of some cases of esophageal cancer treated by XZ-C immune regulation anti-cancer Chinese medicine

6. XZ-C immunoregulatory anti-cancer traditional Chinese medicine for the treatment of esophageal cancer and some cases of cardia cancer

7. List of some cases of XZ-C immunoregulatory anti-cancer Chinese medicine for breast cancer treatment

8. XZ-C immune regulation anti-cancer Chinese medicine treatment of colorectal cancer, a list of some cases

9. List of some cases of XZ-C immunoregulatory anti-cancer Chinese medicine for treatment of cholangiocarcinoma

Part II

XZ-C Immunoregulation Anti-cancer Traditional Chinese Medicine Treating Typical Cases of Malignant Tumor

1. Treatment of some typical cases of liver cancer

2. Some typical cases of postoperative adjuvant treatment of pancreatic cancer

3. Some typical cases of adjuvant treatment after gastric cancer

4. some typical cases of postoperative adjuvant treatment of lung cancer

5. Typical cases of adjuvant treatment after esophageal cancer

6. Typical cases of adjuvant treatment after breast cancer surgery

7. Some typical cases of adjuvant treatment after rectal cancer

8. Some typical cases of postoperative adjuvant treatment of gallbladder cancer

9. Some typical cases of postoperative adjuvant treatment such as kidney cancer and bladder cancer

10. Some typical cases of postoperative adjuvant treatment such as thyroid cancer and retroperitoneal tumors

11. Some typical cases of non-Hodgkin's lymphoma treatment

12. A typical case of chemotherapy + XZ-C Chinese medicine in the treatment of acute lymphoblastic leukemia

Part II

Typical Cases of XZ-C Immunoregulation Anti-cancer Traditional Chinese Medicine Treating Malignant Tumor

1. Some typical cases of Treatment of liver cancer

Case 1

Mao xxx, male, 48 years old, cadre, Tianmen. Medical record number: xxxx

Diagnosis:

Primary liver cancer

Fig. Diagnosis and treatment of primary liver cancer

1994.8.11	1994.8.30	1994 11.26	1995	1996.12	1997	1998	Continue taking medication	2010.5
B ultrasound	surgery	XZ-C	XZ-C	surgery	XZ-C	XZ-C	⟶	XZ-C
PHC								

Taking XZ-C1+4+5

Medical history and treatment:

On August 1, 1994, due to exhaustion and fatigue, he went to the local county hospital for a B-ultrasound, and found a 4.1cmX4.5cm space-occupying lesion in the left liver.

On May 26, 1994, the left hepatic lobe was resectioned in Union Hospital.

Pathological section: hepatocellular carcinoma, without other treatment.

After the operation, the patient came to the $XZ-C_{1+4+5}$ anti-cancer immune Chinese medicine treatment at the outpatient department of the Integrated Chinese and Western Anti-cancer Cooperation Group. After taking the medicine, the spirit, appetite and physical strength were restored.

The patient has been taking XZ-C immune traditional Chinese medicine for a long time, and the patient came to the outpatient clinic for check-ups and medicines every month. The general condition is good and the patient has resumed work.

By the B-ultrasound re-examination on December 14, 1996, it was found that the left extrahepatic lobe had a space-occupying lesion about 1.3cm X 1.8cm in size. The left extrahepatic lobe was resectioned in Union Hospital on December 30, 1996. Continue XZ-C1+4+5 anti-relapse and anti-metastasis immune Chinese medicine treatment.

At the time of the return visit, the patient continued to take XZ-C Chinese medicine for a long time without interruption.

In May 2010, the patient returned for a follow-up visit. The general condition is good, the complexion is rosy, the body is strong, and the normal person is healthy, and he has resumed physical work for 11 years. The spirit and appetite are good. Daily the patient eats 600g food. Re-examination of B-ultrasound showed no abnormalities. See picture 1.

Evaluation:

This patient underwent left hepatic lobectomy on August 26, 1994 due to a 4.1cmx 4.5cm space-occupying lesion in the left liver, and was treated with XZ-C immunoregulatory Chinese medicine after the operation.

On December 30, 1996, the left liver was found to have another 1.3cm x 1.8cm space-occupying lesions were resectioned on the left lateral lobules, followed by XZ-C traditional Chinese medicine treatment, long-term $XZ-C_{1+4+5}$, 16 years of follow-up visits, good health, and years of returning to physical work.

This example prompts:

After liver cancer resection, take XZ-C1+4+5 immunomodulatory Chinese medicine for a long time, protect Thymus and increase immune function, protect bone marrow and produce blood, protect the liver function, improve the overall immune function and disease resistance, surgery + XZ-C immune Chinese medicine, which can consolidate the long-term effect after surgery.

Case 2

Liu XXX, female, 65 years old, cadre, Jianshi County,
Hubei Medical Record Number: XXXX

Diagnosis:

Primary massive liver cancer

The figure of Diagnosis and treatment of liver cancer cases:

1995.	1995.	1995.11	1996	1997	1998	1999	2000	2001	2002	2003	2004	2005
7.4	7.11	Intervention										
CT	XZ-C	One time	XZ-C	XZ-C	XZ-C	XZ-C	XZ-C	XZ-C	XZ-C	XZ-C	XZ-C	XZ-C

Primary massive
liver cancer

Serve XZ-C1+4+5

Medical history and treatment:

Due to upper abdominal discomfort for half a month, CT was performed at Union Hospital on July 4, 1995. The examination reported that there was a 6.7cmX7.1cmX9cm space-occupying lesion in the right lobe of the liver, which was confirmed to be primary liver cancer.

He did not want surgery or chemotherapy. He started taking XZ-C1+5 treatment at the outpatient clinic of the Integrative Chinese and Western Anticancer Cooperation Group on July 11, 1995. After 2 months, his spirit and appetite improved significantly, and he gained weight. On September 20, 1995, the CT mass was smaller than before.

Interventional embolization was done once in November 1995, and no other treatments have been used since.

I have been taking XZ-C traditional Chinese medicine for more than 6 years, and I have been in good health for 10 years. After follow-up in May 2005, the general condition is good and the health is like a normal elderly person. See picture above.

Analysis and evaluation:

This patient was diagnosed as primary liver cancer by CT examination on July 4, 1995. He was treated with XZ-C Chinese medicine one week later, and CT reported that the tumor had shrunk two months later. On November 21, 1995, he was embolized once on November 21, 1995. Since then, the patient has been taking XZ-C Chinese medicine alone, and it has been 10 years since I am as healthy as ordinary people.

This example prompts:

Intervention + XZ-C immune traditional Chinese medicine has a good effect on liver cancer. Intervention can embolize the blood supply of the artery of the cancer focus, and chemotherapy can kill some cancer cells in the cancer focus.

After TAB in most liver cancers, there are still surviving cancer cells in and under the envelope of the tumor.

Due to incomplete necrosis of the tumor, collateral circulation is quickly obtained and continues to grow.

XZ-C immune regulation Chinese medicine can protect the thymus gland and improve immunity, protect the marrow and produce blood, and improve the overall immune function.

Moreover, 85% of liver cancer patients are on the basis of liver cirrhosis. TACE chemotherapy drugs have certain damage to the liver.

XZ-C Chinese medicine can protect liver function, and the combination of intervention + XZ-C immune Chinese medicine can achieve both. Inhibit the tumor and protect the host, both to eliminate the association and strengthen the body, thereby consolidating and maintaining the long-term effect.

Case 3

Ke xxx, male, 54 years old, cadre in Yangxin,
Hubei Medical record number: xxxxx

Diagnosis

Primary liver cancer

The Figure of Diagnosis and treatment of primary liver cancer:

1998.8	PHC 1998.9	1998.9 XZ-C	1998. 10 Pump chemotherapy	1999 XZ-C	2000 XZ-C	2001 XZ-C	2002 XZ-C

Surgical   pump

Exploration   chemotherapy

Liver A   taking XZ-Cl+4+5

Intubation

Medical history and treatment:

Her right upper abdomen was painful for half a month and her appetite lost. CT examination at Yangxin County Hospital found that the right anterior lobe, right posterior lobe, and left inner lobe occupying lesions.

It was to diagnose primary liver cancer. Laparotomy was performed on August 20, 1998. During the operation, the main tumor was found at the hilar of the liver. Both left and right livers had metastases and could not be resected. A chemotherapy pump was used in the hepatic artery. The postoperative treatment was performed once and both Cisplatin + Adriamycin were injected into the pump.

For the second chemotherapy in October 1998, carboplatin + adriamycin was injected through a pump. The pump was not used again because it was blocked.

On September 8, 1998, the patient came to the outpatient clinic of the Anti-cancer Research Cooperation Group of Integrated Traditional Chinese and Western Medicine and treated with Chinese medicine XZ-Cl+4+5.

After taking the medicine for 1 month, the patient has a good appetite, weight gain, ruddy complexion, a soft abdomen, no liver and spleen, generally in good condition, completely take care of my life, and take a long-distance bus from Yangxin to Wuhan clinic every month to take the medicine for review. The patient felt no discomfort, and there was no abnormality in the physical examination.

When the patient came to the outpatient clinic for follow-up visit on June 4, 2002, he was generally in good condition, with a ruddy complexion, walking, moving, talking and laughing like normal healthy people, and no abnormalities in the physical examination. Seeing the figure above.

Analysis and evaluation:

CT of this patient found space-occupying lesions in the anterior, posterior, and left inner lobe of the liver. On August 20, 1998, a laparotomy revealed that the liver cancer had metastasized to both the left and right livers and could not be resected. A chemotherapy pump was installed. He was treated twice with chemotherapy. On September 8, 1998, he came to the outpatient clinic of the cooperative group to use XZ-C 1+4+5 immunomodulatory Chinese medicine treatment. By the end of 2002, he was in good health and no distant metastasis occurred.

This example prompts:

When liver cancer cannot be resected through laparotomy, a chemotherapy pump can be placed in the hepatic artery, and XZ-C1+4+5 immunoregulatory Chinese medicine treatment can be used after the operation to protect the thymus, bone marrow, and liver, improve overall immune function, and induce the body to produce anti-cancer factors in order to control cancer foci, tumor development can be controlled.

Case 4

Qi xxxx, male, 51 years old, cadre, Yingcheng, Hubei
Case number: xxxxx

Diagnosis:

Primary liver cancer

The Figure of Diagnosis and treatment of primary liver cancer is as the following:

1997.10.30　　1997.11.25　　1998　　1999　　1999. 11 2002　2002. 6

CT diagnosis　XZ-C1+4+5　XZ-C　XZ-C　XZ-C　　XZ-C Died after surgery in a foreign hospital

B ultrasound

Diagnose　　Take XZ-C1, XZ-C4, XZ-C5XZ-C Chinese Medicine. No radiotherapy or

liver cancer　chemotherapy, basically recovered

Medical history and treatment:

A CT examination on October 30, 1997 found that the left liver occupies a size of 4.6cmX 3.6cm, and the right lobe of the liver occupies a size of 1.6cmX 1.6cm. The report was: Liver cancer.

Color Doppler ultrasound in Union Hospital on November 11, 1997:

The left liver lobe 5.9cm X 4.0cm X 5.4cm occupies the space, the right liver lobe 2.lcmX1.8crn occupies the space;

Hepatic angiography report: liver cancer.

HBsAg(+), AFP(-).

Due to poor liver function, surgery and intervention are not possible.

Drinking history for 40 years, one meal is about 250ml, he suffered from hepatitis B in 1996 and schistosomiasis in 1966.

On November 25, 1997, he came to the Anti-Cancer Collaborative Group for combined treatment with Chinese and Western medicine;

And he started to take XZ-C1, XZ-C4, XZ-C5. In 1998 and 1999, this patient came to Wulu outpatient clinic from Yingcheng County for review and medicine every month.

The patient is in good condition, ruddy, talking and laughing as usual.

The follow-up visit on November 2, 1999 showed that the liver B-ultrasound lesions were significantly reduced.

The patient can be engaged in light physical work without discomfort. For more than 2 years, the patient has been taking XZ-C1+4+5 without interruption. After consciously taking the medicine, the patient has good appetite and good physical strength.

At the beginning of June 2002, the patient was introduced to Beijing xxx General Hospital for medical treatment (before the patient went to Beijing, my condition was generally good, and my walking activities were normal).

In the hospital for surgical exploration, there was a liver cancer mass of about 5cm X 6cm during the operation, which was the same as the onset 5 years ago. There were tumor thrombi in the bile duct, no metastasis in the abdominal cavity, no ascites, no intrahepatic metastasis, but the tumor was close to the hepatic portal and difficult to remove, it was still to take the bile duct tumor thrombus out and put T tube drainage. After the operation, there was no urine, acute renal failure, and death 6 days after the operation. See the above figure.

Analysis and evaluation:

CT of the patient found on October 30, 1997, that the left liver had an occupying lesion of 4. 6cmX 3. 6cm. On November 11, 1997, the right lobe of the liver was found to occupy 2.1cmX1.8cm. Due to poor liver function, he could not be operated or intervened. There is no other treatment which was used.

The XZ-C1+4+5 immunomodulatory treatment has been used for more than 5 years in the outpatient clinic of the Anti-Cancer Cooperation Group on November 25, 1997, and the health condition is good.

The treatment experience of this patient is:

XZ-C Chinese medicine improves the overall immune function of the host (cellular and humoral immune function), protects the central and surrounding immune organs, protects the liver and kidneys, induces tumor suppressor factors, stabilizes cancer foci, and prevents metastasis and spread.

XZ-C Chinese medicine is a non-damaging treatment, **sincerely for strengthening the body to eliminate evil, and the patient's mental state is good, which is conducive to defeating the disease and conducive to recovery, thus achieving better curative effects.**

This patient was in stable condition after taking XZ-C Chinese medicine for 5 years. The liver cancer has not increased or metastasized. He is generally in good condition and has no discomfort. He walks, talks and laughs as normal.

During my visit to Beijing for treatment this time, XXX General Hospital was diagnosed with hepatocellular carcinoma by surgical exploration and pathology. The tumor was in the hilar of the liver and could not be removed. Because of the bile duct tumor thrombus, the tumor thrombus was taken and T tube drainage was performed. The patient has been anuria after the operation and died of acute renal failure. If the liver and kidney are not attacked by surgical exploration, this may not necessarily be the case. It is a pity!

Case 5

Huang xxx, 53 years old, male, from Wuhan City Medical record number: xxxx

Diagnosis:

Primary massive liver cancer, post-hepatitis cirrhosis, advanced schistosomiasis, portal hypertension

The figure of the diagnosis and treatment of primary liver cancer is as the following:

2000.9	2000 10.19	2001 1.2	2001 3.31	2001 11.12	2002. 1.9	2003	2004	2005
CT Intervention	Intervene	Intervene	intervention	Intervene	XZ-C	XZ-C	XZ-C	XZ-C

Right liver

13.6cmx11.8 cm   Intervention   XZ-C

Occupy

Medical history and treatment:

In September 2000, due to anorexia and abdominal discomfort, the Finance and Trade Hospital had a CT examination:

Right liver 13. 6cmX 11.8cm low-density round lesions.

On September 7th of the same year, I went to Xiehe Hospital for MRI examination:

A huge space-occupying lesion of 13.1cmX11.4cmX12.5cm was seen in the right lobe of the liver.

It was diagnosed at Union Hospital on September 13 as:

Massive liver cancer in the right lobe of the liver.

It was to do the right hepatic artery infusion chemotherapy + embolization.

The second hepatic artery chemoembolization was performed on October 19, 2000;

For the third time on January 2, 2001:

The fourth time on March 30, 2001:

It was the fifth time on November 12, 2001.

Interventional chemotherapy medication is HCPT 25mg+5-FU 1000mg, lipiodol 10ml+MMC 10mg.

The current situation is generally good.

The lesion changes after intervention are as follows:

On October 12, 2000, CT examination of the right lobe of the liver lesion 11.1cmX11.8cm;

On December 4, 2000, CT examination of the right lobe of the liver lesion was 10.8cmX9.8cm. The lesion was basically stable and reduced.

In February 2001, CT examination of the right lobe of the liver lesion

10. 5cmX9.5cm;

On September 3, 2001, CT examination of the right liver lobe lesion was 9.8cmX8. The 9cm lesion was basically stable and reduced to some extent.

On January 9, 2001, I came to Shuguang Oncology Specialty Clinic to take XZ-C immunomodulatory Chinese medicine XZ-C1+4+5 for treatment. After taking the medicine, the general condition is good, and the spirit, appetite and sleep are good.

The patient comes to the outpatient clinic for follow-up visits every month to take XZ-C1+4+5 immunomodulatory Chinese medicine. The condition of the follow-up visit on October 21, 2002 is stable, with good general condition, good spirits, appetite, urine and bowel as usual, normal walking activities, and good health recovery.

B-ultrasound and CT re-examination of the lesions are the same as before, doing housework in the morning, playing cards in the afternoon, living a regular life, regular exercise, never caught a cold, follow-up visits for 4 and a half years, like healthy elderly, good quality of life, no discomfort. See the above figure.

Analysis and evaluation:

This case is a primary massive liver cancer. After 5 interventions, the cancer focus has been reduced and good results have been achieved. The last intervention was on November 12, 2001. At this time, the right lobe of the liver was 9.8cmX8. 9cm, started to take XZ-C1+4+5 treatment at the Shuguang Oncology Clinic on January 96, 2002.

XZ-C1 can kill cancer cells, but not normal cells;

XZ-C4 protects the thymus, prevents thymus atrophy, and improves immunity;

XZ-C5 protects the liver and has been taking XZ-C Chinese medicine daily for 3 years.

It has been 4 and a half years by the time of the follow-up visit. The condition is generally good and the condition is stable without metastasis or development.

The patient has good spirits, good appetite, regular walking activities.

The treatment experience of this case is:

Interventional therapy is first used for massive liver cancer to shrink and stabilize the cancer focus, and then take XZ-C immunomodulatory Chinese medicine to consolidate the long-term effect, protect the liver, increase immunity, and control blood metastasis.

Case 6

Li xxx, Male, 53 years old, a farmer from Caidian,
Wuhan Medical record number: xxxxxx

Diagnosis:

Primary massive liver cancer, advanced schistosomiasis cirrhosis

The figure of the therapy course of massive primary liver cancer is as the following:

2001	2001.	2002	2003	2004	2005
03.01	03.09	XZ-C	XZ-C	XZ-C	XZ-C

⟶

Laparotomy   XZ-C1+4+5

Medical history and treatment:

On January 22, 2001, he felt pain in his right back and back.

On February 26, the B-ultrasound found a lump in the liver,

On January 31, 2001, CT showed a 14cm×1cm space-occupying lesion in the right lobe of the liver, which was diagnosed as massive liver cancer in the right lobe.

An exploratory laparotomy was performed at Tongji Hospital on March 1. The tumor was too large to be resected, and a drug pump was placed in the portal vein.

After the operation, the drug pump is injected once (mitomycin and 5-FU).

The patient has a history of schistosomiasis for 30 years.

On March 9, 2001, he came to Shuguang Tumor Specialist Clinic to take XZ-C immunoregulatory Chinese medicine treatment.

Use XZ-C1+4+5, LMS, MDZ, and apply XZ-C3 externally to the large fist mass under the right costal margin.

After taking the medicine for 1 month, her general condition improved, her spirit and appetite improved, and the mass under the costal margin of her right upper abdomen became soft and shrunk.

After taking the medicine for 3 months, the general condition is good, the appetite and sleep are good, the physical strength is gradually restored, and the walking activities are as normal.

Re-examination of B-ultrasound on October 22, 2001:

See 6cmX7.8cm occupancy on the right lobe of liver, continue to take XZ-C1+4+5 treatment and XZ-C3 external application,

A comprehensive review on November 19, 2003 showed that the intrahepatic lesions in B-ultrasound were the same as before, the kidneys were not abnormal, the chest radiographs were not abnormal, the subclavian lymph nodes were buckled, and the right subcostal mass was significantly reduced, soft, with clear borders. Pain, continue to take XZ-C1+4+5. See the above figure.

Analysis and evaluation:

This patient had a massive liver cancer, which could not be removed by surgical exploration, and was given 1 chemotherapy session with a drug pump in the portal vein. The patient started to come to the clinic in March 2001 to take the Chinese medicine XZ-C1+4+5 for immune regulation and control anticancer and XZ-C3 for external application. The medication has been persisted for 4 years, the disease condition is stable, has not continued to develop, and has not been transferred.

Case 7

Wang xxx, male, 40 years old, teacher,Shandong,
Medical record number: xxxx

Diagnosis:

Hepatocellular carcinoma

The Figure of Diagnosis and treatment of hepatocellular carcinoma is as the following:

1989.6	1995.2	1995.6	1995. 11	1995. 12	1995. 12	1996 1997 1998 1999
Thymoma	CT	intervention	Right liver	relapse	XZ-C	
Resection Liver	cancer	once	Excision	Metastatic lung	traditional Chinese medicine	

taking XZ-C1+4+5

Medical history and treatment:

On June 28, 1989, he underwent longitudinal tumor resection, pathological section: lymphocytic thymoma, extremely malignant, there is no other treatment.

In February 1995, B-ultrasound was re-examined, and it was found that the liver had occupying lesions.

On February 23, 1995 CT shows :

The posterior segment of the right liver lobe occupies 8.2cmX8.7cm, and multiple nodules are fused.

On June 5, 1995, he underwent liver A radiography + check plug chemotherapy.

The space-occupying lesion remained after interventional treatment, but the right hepatic wedge resection was performed on November 10, 1995.

Pathological section: hepatocellular carcinoma.

B-ultrasound review on December 21, 1995 is as the following:

The 3.8cmX3.2cm occupancy in the right lobe of the liver is a recurrence of liver cancer after surgery, right pleural effusion and right lower lung atelectasis, chest radiograph showing metastasis of right lower lung and liver cancer,

The patients came to the XZ-Cl+4+5 series of anti-cancer escalation Chinese medicine treatment at the outpatient clinic of the Integrated Chinese and Western Anticancer Cooperation Group on December 23, 1995.

The patient has been taking XZ-C Chinese medicine for more than 2 years, and it has been 5 years at the time of return. The general condition is good, the patient was teaching at work, working normally, there is no other treatments. See the above Figure.

Evaluation:

CT of this patient in May 1995 shows: the right lobe of the liver was 7.1cmX6. 6cm, and the interventional embolization was performed once in 1995.

On November 10, 1995, the right liver was excised in a wedge shape and he was hepatocellular carcinoma.

On December 21, 1995, B-ultrasound found a recurrence of the right lobe of the liver 3.8cm X 3.2cm.

On December 23, 1995, he came to the cooperative group XZ-C immune regulation Chinese medicine treatment, and the condition is good, and it has been more than 4 years.

This example prompts:

The comprehensive treatment with liver cancer with interventional embolization + surgical resection + XZ-C immune traditional Chinese medicine can achieve better results.

Case 8

Zhao xxx, Female, 34 years old, Jingzhou, Auditor
Medical record number: xxxx

Diagnosis:

Primary massive liver cancer

The figure of diagnosis and treatment of primary massive liver cancer is as the following:

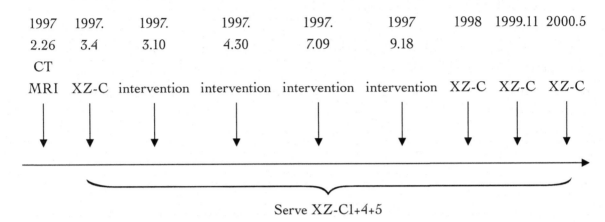

1997	1997.	1997.	1997.	1997.	1997	1998	1999.11	2000.5
2.26	3.4	3.10	4.30	7.09	9.18			
CT								
MRI	XZ-C	intervention	intervention	intervention	intervention	XZ-C	XZ-C	XZ-C

Serve XZ-Cl+4+5

Medical history and treatment:

On February 26, 1997, because the stomach was not suitable for B-ultrasound, it was found that there was a 1.3cmX 10. 4cm space-occupying lesion between the liver side and the left lobe and the MRI was 7.9cm X 11. 2cmX 11. 0cm; it is the portal vein has Cancer thrombus.

The patient had fever since March 1, 390C, transferred to Union Hospital on March 2, still high fever, there was a 5cmX6cm mass, hard in quality on the area of the low part of the xiphoid bone.

Intervention was performed on March 10, and the response was great. Intervention for chemoembolization was performed on April 30,

There was the intervention for the third time on July 9, and intervention for the fourth time on September 18.

The tumor was significantly reduced.

On March 4, 1997, he came to the outpatient clinic of the Integrated Chinese and Western Anticancer Research Cooperation Group to take XZ-Cl+4+5 immunoregulatory Chinese medicine to stabilize the lesion, control the spread and progression, and prevent metastasis.

After taking the XZ-C series of medicines, the spirit and appetite improved significantly, the condition recovered well, and the quality of life was good. The original rib buckle and lumps has not been touched for 2 and a half years. See the above picture.

Evaluation:

This patient with massive liver cancer received 4 interventions and insisted on taking XZ-C immunoregulatory Chinese medicine for a long time. It was interventional + XZ-C Chinese medicine treatment. The effect was good and the quality of life was good. The original rib buckle and lumps have not been found. It has been in good condition for more than 3 years.

This example prompts:

Intervention + XZ-C Chinese medicine has a good comprehensive effect. Intervention kills some cancer cells, and the tumor is significantly reduced, but there are still living cancer cells and continue to proliferate and grow. After intervention, the patient takes XZ-Cl+4+5 immunoregulation Chinese medicine for a long time, XZ-Cl+4 can inhibit 10^5 cancer cells.

Taking XZ-C immune traditional Chinese medicine for a long time can control cancer, stabilize the lesion and prevent metastasis.

A big contradiction in interventional chemotherapy against cancer is:

Cancer cells continue to divide and proliferate, while chemotherapy can only be used intermittently. This is a contradiction. During the intermittent period of chemotherapy, cancer cells will continue to grow. Intervention is a fatal blow to the cancer focus and then long-term use of XZ-C immunomodulatory Chinese medicine, the combination of the two may consolidate the curative effect and maintain a better curative effect for a long time.

Case 9

Zengxxx, Male, 48 years old, cadre, Enshi
Medical record number: xxxx

Diagnosis:

Primary liver cancer

The figure of the diagnosis and treatment of primary liver cancer is as the following:

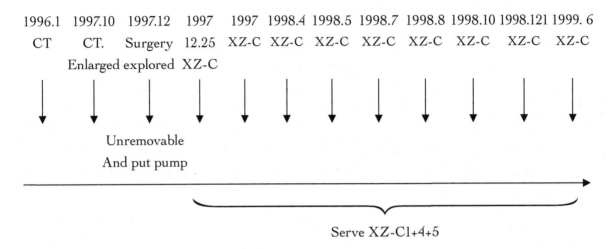

| 1996.1 | 1997.10 | 1997.12 | 1997 | 1997 | 1998.4 | 1998.5 | 1998.7 | 1998.8 | 1998.10 | 1998.121 | 1999. 6 |
| CT | CT. | Surgery | 12.25 | XZ-C | XZ-C | XZ-C | XZ-C | XZ-C | XZ-C | XZ-C | XZ-C |

Enlarged explored XZ-C

Unremovable
And put pump

Serve XZ-C1+4+5

Medical history and treatment:

In January 1996, in Enshi, CT showed that the size of the lesion in the right lobe of the liver was found and was treated with liver protection.

In mid-October 1997, local color Doppler ultrasound revealed that the liver mass was enlarged, 5.7crnX5.7cm; then the patient was hospitalized in the Department of Surgery of Union Hospital in October 1997.

On November 7, 1997, he had an exploratory laparotomy, and he could not be resected. Hepatic artery intubation was performed with pump chemotherapy. Intraoperative tissue section showed: **hepatocellular carcinoma.**

On December 23, 1997, the second hepatic artery pump injection chemotherapy, due to a large response, was not treated again afterwards, and no pump injection was performed.

XZ-C series of immunological regulation and control Chinese medicines have been used in the outpatient clinic of the Anti-Cancer Cooperation Group since December 25, 1997.

After treatment, the general condition was good at the time of the follow-up visit, the mental appetite was good, the physical strength was restored, and the walking activities were normal without discomfort.

The patient returned to work in November, went to work every day, and worked as a teacher at the Tobacco Technical School. He was both mentally and physically competent in teaching class. See the above figure.

Evaluation:

This patient had a CT scan in January 1996 and found a right hepatic lesion. On November 7, 1997, he was unresectable by laparotomy at Xiehe Hospital. He was intubated in the hepatic artery with pump chemotherapy and injected twice. On December 23, 1997 after two injections, there was no chemotherapy. On December 25, 1997, he came to the outpatient clinic with XZ-C1+4+5 immunomodulatory Chinese medicine for nearly 3 years, and the condition is good.

This example prompts:

Hepatic artery intubation pump chemotherapy + XZ-C immunomodulation Chinese medicine treatment has good results. Hepatic artery intubation pump chemotherapy can kill most cells in liver cancer lesions + XZ-C immunomodulation Chinese medicine treatment which can attack and kill cancer cells and protect the host and improve the overall immune function and improve to monitor residual cancer cells, and a better curative effect has been achieved.

Case 10

Wei xxx, Female, 36 years old, from Chibi, Hubei
Medical record number: xxxx

Diagnosis:

Hepatocellular carcinoma

The figure of diagnosis and treatment of hepatocellular carcinoma is as the following:

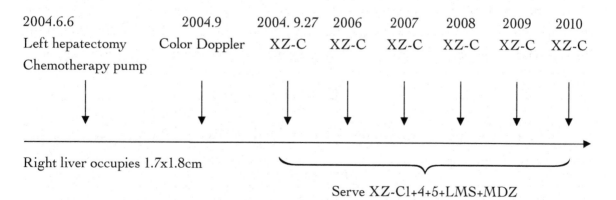

2004.6.6	2004.9	2004. 9.27	2006	2007	2008	2009	2010
Left hepatectomy	Color Doppler	XZ-C	XZ-C	XZ-C	XZ-C	XZ-C	XZ-C
Chemotherapy pump							

Right liver occupies 1.7x1.8cm

Serve XZ-C1+4+5+LMS+MDZ

Medical history and treatment:

Upper abdominal distension and pain, anorexia, fatigue for half a month, CT shows is as: left liver spac-occupied, AFP>400.

On June 6, 2004, a left hepatectomy + portal vein chemotherapy pump was performed at Chibi City People's Hospital. During the operation, the tumor basically occupied the left liver. After the left hepatectomy, the chemotherapy pump was placed in the right gastro-omental vein. (the ending portal vein), chemotherapy was given by pump 2 times after operation. B-ultrasound showed 1.7cm X 1.8cm space in right liver 2 months after operation. Postoperative pathology: fibrolamel hepatocellular carcinoma.

On September 27, 2004, the XZ-C immune-regulated and control anti-cancer Chinese medicine treatment of Mi Shuguang Cancer Specialist Outpatient Clinic, with XZ-C1+4+5, LMS and MDZ, came to the outpatient clinic for follow-up visits every month and kept taking the medicine.

Liver color Doppler ultrasound was reviewed in the outpatient clinic on April 8, 2008. There is no abnormality which was found. AFP returned to normal.

He is generally in good condition, with good mental appetite, weight gain, good physical strength, and even working in Wenzhou, with good health. He has been taking medicine for seven years and is in good health. See the above figure.

Analysis and evaluation:

This patient received chemotherapy pump in ten portal vein after left hepatic cancer and left hepatectomy. He received chemotherapy twice with drug pump. He came to the clinic to take xz-c immunoregulatory Chinese medicine for a long time. The patient has been taking a small amount of medicine for a long time for 7 years, and the patient's health has recovered well. The patient has been working in Wenzhou for the past three years, sending medicine every month, and my condition is good.

Case 11

Huangxxx, Male,38yo, Hubei Worker Medical Record Number: xxxx

Diagnosis:

Primary liver cancer surgery

The figure of postoperative diagnosis and treatment of primary liver cancer is as the following:

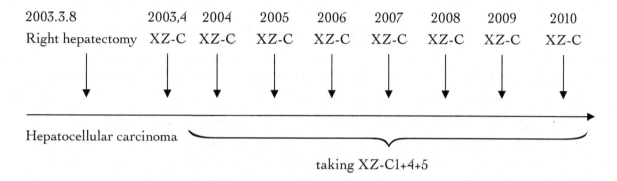

Hepatocellular carcinoma

taking XZ-C1+4+5

Medical history and treatment:

On February 16, 2003, a liver tumor was found by B-ultrasound due to a physical examination on February 16, 2003. CT report showed that the right posterior lower lobe of the liver was 9.8X5.6 cm and the boundary between the normal liver parenchyma and the normal liver parenchyma was blurred. It was a massive liver cancer.

He underwent right hepatectomy at Union Hospital on March 8, 2003. Postoperative pathology:

Hepatocellular carcinoma.

Because of financial difficulties, he did not receive chemotherapy, so he came to Shuguang Oncology Specialty Clinic to take XZ-C immunomodulatory postoperative adjuvant treatment.

Treated with XZ-C1+4+5, the patient insisted on taking XZ-C4+5 for a long time, and came to an outpatient clinic every 2 months. It has been 8 years so far. The general condition is good. It has been 4 years since the patient resumed carpentry work and is competent without discomfort.

On December 10, 2009, he came to the outpatient clinic for follow-up visits and medicine. The general condition was good, the appetite was good, and there was no discomfort.

This year, the patient came to Wuhan from Hefei, Anhui (workplace) for review. The general condition is good and my health is good. Due to financial difficulties, the patient could not undergo chemotherapy after surgery and took XZ-C4+5 alone. It has been 8 years so far. See the above picture.

Analysis and evaluation:

This patient is hepatocellular carcinoma. After right hepatectomy, due to financial difficulties, he did not receive chemotherapy. After the operation, XZ-C1+4+5 immunoregulatory Chinese medicine was used as postoperative adjuvant treatment, and he insisted on taking XZ-C immunity for a long time. It has been more than 8 years since it has been more than 8 years and 4 years since it has resumed work.

This example prompts:

XZ-C immunomodulatory Chinese medicine can be used as an adjuvant treatment after liver cancer resection, which can improve the overall immune function to prevent recurrence and metastasis.

Case 12

Li xxx, Male, 60-year-old, Wuhan, cadre
Medical record number: xxxx

Diagnosis:

Hepatocellular carcinoma

The figure of diagnosis and treatment of hepatocellular carcinoma is as the following:

2005.11	2005.11.28	2006	2007	2008	2009	2010
Right hepatectomy	XZ-C	XZ-C	XZ-C	XZ-C	XZ-C	XZ-C

Hepatocellular carcinoma

Serve XZ-C, LMS+MDZ

Medical history and treatment:

Physical examination in November 2005, B-ultrasound found that the right lobe of the liver was 5.4cm X 4.0cm2 occupying the space. He was resected on the right hepatectomy in Wuhan Third Hospital in November 2005. Postoperative pathology: hepatocellular carcinoma.

No chemotherapy was given after the operation.

On November 28, 2005, the patient came to Shuguang Oncology Clinic to use XZ-C immunomodulatory anti-cancer Chinese medicine as postoperative adjuvant treatment, and took XZ-C1+4+5+LMS+M DZ to protect Thymus and increase the immune function, to protect bone marrow to produce blood.

The patient come to the outpatient clinic for follow-up visits and picks up medicines every month. The patient has been taking medicine for a long time for 5 years. The general condition is good, the appetite is good, and the health condition is good. See the above picture.

Analysis and evaluation:

The patient's physical examination found that hepatic space was occupied. He had undergone a right hepatectomy. No chemotherapy was given after the operation. He took XZ-C immunomodulatory anticancer Chinese medicine as an adjuvant treatment after the operation. Long-term medication has been persisted. It has been 5 years and the patient is in good health.

2. **Some typical cases of postoperative adjuvant treatment of <u>pancreatic cancer</u>**

Case 13

Yao xxx, Female, 73 years old, Wuhan
Medical record number: xxxx

Diagnosis:

Postoperative papillary adenocarcinoma of the gallbladder

The figure of the course of treatment after papillary adenocarcinoma of the gallbladder is as the following:

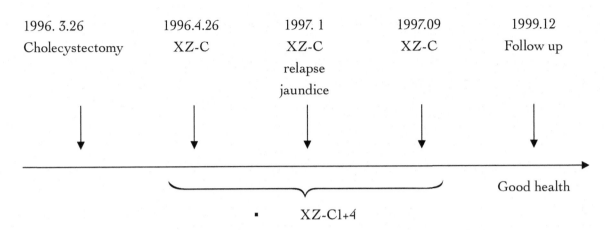

Medical history and treatment:

The right subcostal pain started at the end of December 1995. The pain intensified in February 1996. He lived in Xiehe Hospital.

On March 26, 1996 he was diagnosed as gallbladder cancer with cholecystectomy + common bile duct T-tube drainage. Pathological report: Papillary adenocarcinoma of the gallbladder invaded the muscular layer of the gallbladder wall, with gallbladder stones.

The T-shaped tube was pulled out on April 26, 1996, and he came to the outpatient clinic of the Integrated Chinese and Western Medicine Anticancer Research Cooperation Group on April 26, 1996, and used XZ-C1+4 immunomodulatory Chinese medicine treatment.

Colic recurred again on January 23, 1997. He was diagnosed with recurrence and obstruction of the lower part of the common bile on B-ultrasound in Xiehe Hospital. The whole body was jaundiced and the common bile duct was dilated by 1.5cm.

2 months after taking XZ-C1+4 Chinese medicine, the jaundice gradually subsided and the mental appetite improved.

The patient continued to take XZ-C1+4 immunoregulatory Chinese medicine for 15 months, and took the medicine on time every month. By July 1997, the patient's condition was completely improved, the spirit and physical strength were restored, and the walking activities were normal. The patient can do housework.

On December 4, 1999, his son came to the clinic for follow-up:

The patient is in good condition after taking XZ-Cl+4 Chinese medicine for one and a half years. He has not taken any medicine in the past two years. He is in good condition and has recovered physical strength. He is doing housework at home, shopping for vegetables and playing cards, just like other healthy grandma. See the above picture.

Evaluation:

This patient underwent cholecystectomy due to gallbladder cancer on March 26, 1996, and was unable to undergo chemotherapy due to old age and infirmity. No other treatment was given. He came to the cooperative group outpatient clinic on April 26, 1996 to be treated with XZ-Cl+4 immunoregulatory Chinese medicine.

In January 1997, he had obstructive jaundice, which gradually subsided after taking XZ-C Chinese medicine for 2 months. The patient insisted on taking XZ-Cl+4 for a long time after the operation, and it had been 4 years at the time of follow-up visit, and he was in good health.

This example prompts:

After gallbladder cancer surgery, the patient is taking XZ-C 14 immunoregulatory Chinese medicine for a longer period of time which can improve the quality of life, prevent recurrence and metastasis, and significantly prolong survival.

Case 14

Zhu XX, male, 53 years old, cadre, Xiaogan
Medical record number: xxxx

Diagnosis:

Pancreatic head adenocarcinoma

The figure of diagnosis and treatment of pancreatic head adenocarcinoma is as the following:

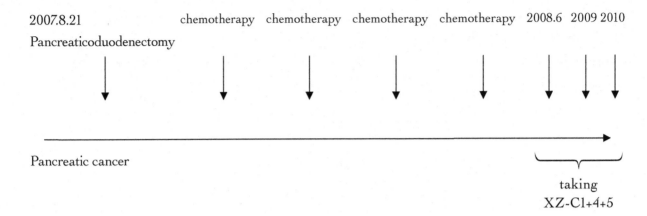

2007.8.21   chemotherapy   chemotherapy   chemotherapy   chemotherapy   2008.6   2009 2010
Pancreaticoduodenectomy

Pancreatic cancer

taking
XZ-Cl+4+5

Medical history and treatment:

CT examination at Xiaogan Hospital due to "jaundice hepatitis" on August 15, 2007: pancreatic head occupation, bile duct obstruction, transferred to Xiehe Hospital. And the patient had pancreaticoduodenectomy on August 21, 2007, postoperative Pathology: Well-differentiated adenocarcinoma involved the pancreas of the common bile duct and the full-thickness of the intestinal wall. The posterior edge of the pancreas and the peritoneum showed cancer tissue involvement. There was no cancer metastasis in the peripancreatic lymph nodes (5 pieces).

After the operation, the patient had chemotherapy for four cycles, WBC decreased, PLT decreased, and toxic side effects were obvious.

The patient came to Shuguang Oncology Clinic on June 16, 2008 to use XZ-Cl+4+5, LMS and MDZ immunomodulation therapy.

After taking the medicine, the general condition is good, and the spirit and appetite are good. I come to the clinic for review and medicine every month. So far, it has been 4 years. The patient came to the outpatient clinic for follow-up visit in September 2010. The condition is generally good, the supraclavicular is not buckled and abnormal, the abdomen is flat and soft, not abnormal, and the incision scar is hyperplastic. The patient has resumed work for one year and doesn't any discomfort. See the above figure.

Analysis and evaluation:

This patient underwent pancreaticoduodenectomy for pancreatic cancer. He was treated with gemcitabine chemotherapy for 4 cycles after the operation. The toxicity was obvious. He came to Shuguang Cancer Specialist Clinic to be treated with XZ-C immunomodulatory Chinese medicine for nearly 4 years. In good condition, work has resumed.

This example prompts:

After pancreatic cancer surgery, XZ-C immune-regulated Chinese medicine is used to protect breasts and promote blood, which is an adjuvant treatment after surgery, which can control metastasis and long-term survival.

Case 15

Fang XXX, Male, 50 years old, farmer from Luotian, Hubei Medical record number: xxxx

Diagnosis:

after exploration of pancreatic head cancer

The figure of the course of diagnosis and treatment of pancreatic cancer as the following:

1996. 11	1996.12	1997	1998	1999	2000	2001
	XZ-C	XZ-C	XZ-C	XZ-C	XZ-C	XZ-C

Surgical exploration pathological section pancreatic cancer

XZ-C

Medical history and treatment:

The upper abdomen was uncomfortable for 3 months.

On November 28, 1996, he had a laparotomy for jaundice in the local hospital: stones were seen in the biliary tract during the operation, and the pancreatic head was enlarged and could not be removed. The pathology of the sample was pancreatic cancer.

Postoperative CT diagnosis: pancreatic head with dilatation of intrahepatic bile duct.

The postoperative jaundice continued and did not go away. The patient came to Shuguang Oncology Clinic to take XZ-C Chinese medicine for immunotherapy on December 11, 1996.

After taking the medicine for 1 month, the general condition improved, and the spirit and appetite improved.

When she was discharged from the hospital, she still had jaundice and excessive sweating. After continuing to take XZ-C medicine and Shugan Lidan Tuihuang Decoction for 2 months, the jaundice gradually subsided and the pain eased.

Four months later, the jaundice disappeared, the spirit was good, the appetite was good, and the abdomen still had slight pain.

By July 1998, he resumed work, participated in light labor, and his face was full of red light. In the past few years, he continued to take XZ-C traditional Chinese medicine, and his health has recovered well.

On April 6, 2004, the patient's family brought another patient to the outpatient clinic. They said that the elderly Fang XX was in good health, walked as usual and could do housework, just like a normal healthy elderly. See the above figure.

Analysis and evaluation:

This patient had pancreatic head cancer and jaundice. He was unresectable by laparotomy on November 28, 1996. Postoperative diagnosis is pancreatic head cancer with dilatation of intrahepatic bile ducts.

The patient came to the clinic on December 11, 1996. After long-term use of XZ-C immune regulation and control anti-cancer medicine and Shugan Lidan Tuihuang Decoction, the jaundice gradually resolved after 7 months, and continued to take XZ-C 1+4 daily for a long time to increase immunity Until July 1998, the patient recovered well.

<u>Taking XZ-C immune regulation and anti-cancer Chinese medicine can soothe the liver and promote gallbladder, strengthen the body, promote blood circulation and remove blood stasis.</u>

After taking the medicine continuously for more than 4 years, it was changed to intermittent medicine for maintenance to consolidate the curative effect. It has been 9 years since the follow-up visit and the patient's health condition is still good.

3. Some typical cases of adjuvant treatment after gastric cancer

Case 16

Cai XX, male, 65 years old, retired cadre Wuhan

Medical record number: xxxx

Diagnosis:

Poorly differentiated adenocarcinoma of the fundus of the stomach, recurrence after radical resection, recurrent cancer of the remnant stomach

The figure of Diagnosis and treatment of recurrent cancer after radical gastric cancer is as the following:

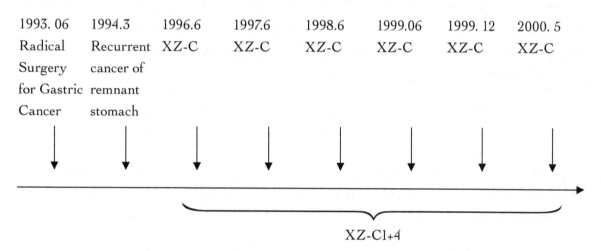

1993. 06	1994.3	1996.6	1997.6	1998.6	1999.06	1999. 12	2000. 5
Radical Surgery for Gastric Cancer	Recurrent cancer of remnant stomach	XZ-C	XZ-C	XZ-C	XZ-C	XZ-C	XZ-C

XZ-C1+4

Medical history and treatment:

The patient had epigastric pain for 1 year. After the diagnosis of gastric cancer, he underwent a radical proximal gastrectomy at Union Hospital in June 1993.

FM chemotherapy was performed once after the operation. Due to anemia, the body was weak and unable to undergo chemotherapy, WBC 1900.

Eight months after the operation, the pain under the xiphoid process was accompanied by vomiting, and the left upper abdomen had been painful for half a year.

On March 25, 1994, he went to the barium meal of Xiehe Hospital: the upper end of the remnant stomach was irregularly filled with defects, part of the mucosa was damaged, and the anastomosis narrowed. The conclusion of the barium meal is: recurrent cancer in the remnant stomach.

B-ultrasound on May 3, 1996: No space-occupying lesions in the liver.

Because the patient cannot eat rice, he can eat half-liquid juice and noodles.

The patient felt tired, weak, mentally ill, and reluctant to undergo another operation.

In June 1996, XZ-C series of immunological Chinese medicines were used in the outpatient clinic of the Combination of Chinese and Western Medicine Anti-cancer Cooperation Group.

After taking the drug, the general condition of the patient improved, and the spirit and appetite improved. He has taken XZ-C daily for more than 4 years.

At the follow-up visit on May 6, 2000, the patient was generally in good condition, with a ruddy complexion, good appetite, talking and laughing, walking as usual, eating porridge and steamed buns for a long time, and was a healthy old man. See the above figure.

Evaluation:

This patient was treated with XZ-C1+4 immune regulation and control traditional Chinese medicine after radical gastric cancer surgery in June 1993 and recurred in the remnant stomach in March 1994.

He has been treated with XZ-C1+4 immune traditional Chinese medicine without other treatment. It has been 6 years and 2 months and he has recovered in good condition.

This example prompts:

Recurrent cancer in the remnant stomach, and the anastomosis is not completely obstructed. The patient can still eat. The XZ-C14 immune regulation and control chinese medicine protect Thymus and increase immune function and can improve the overall immune function, which can control the tumor to and prevent its development, prevent metastasis, stabilize the lesion, and make the condition improve significantly and the patient can live and survive for a long time.

Case 17

Liu XXX, 65 years old Wuhan economist

Medical record number: xxxx

Diagnosis:

Gastric Fundus Cancer

The figure of diagnosis and treatment of adenocarcinoma in the stomach is as the following:

1995.1	1996.3	1997	1997.8	1999	2000	2001	2002	2003
Surgery	XZ-C	XZ-C	XZ-C	XZ-C	XZ-C	XZ-C	XZ-C	XZ-C

XZ-Cl+4

Medical history and treatment:

In January 1995, due to stomach pain for half a year, it was confirmed by gastroscopy that the patient had hilar adenocarcinoma which was a radical gastrectomy, proximal gastrectomy, and esophagogastric anastomosis.

The postoperatively was fine, due to poor physical strength and weight loss, it was not suitable for chemotherapy.

The patient came to the Integrative Chinese and Western Medicine Anti-Cancer Collaborative Group on March 16, 1996 for the treatment of biological immune traditional Chinese medicine. The patient used XZ-Cl+4 immunotherapy alone and continued XZ- C drug was used for 5 years, and the intermittent medication was generally in good condition. No other treatment was used after the operation. See the above figure.

Analysis and evaluation:

This patient had a proximal gastrectomy and gastroesophageal anastomosis for cancer of the fundus of the stomach in January 1995, and due to be frailty and the body thin, chemotherapy is not suitable, and XZ-C1+4 immune traditional Chinese medicine has been used for more than 10 years after the operation. The general condition is good.

This example prompts:

XZ-C immuno-regulatory and control anti-cancer Chinese medicine can prevent recurrence and metastasis after surgery, and the effect is better.

Case 18

Chen XX, male, 65 years old worker Wuhan
Medical record number: xxxx

Diagnosis:

Postoperative recurrence and metastasis of gastric cancer

The figure of Diagnosis and treatment of recurrence and metastasis of gastric cancer after surgery is as the following:

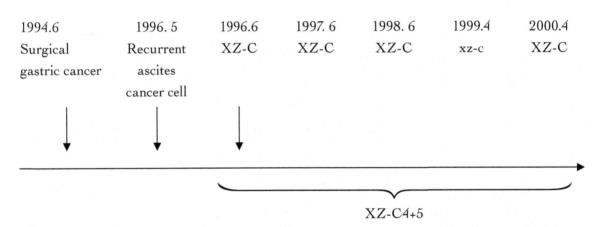

1994.6	1996. 5	1996.6	1997. 6	1998. 6	1999.4	2000.4
Surgical	Recurrent	XZ-C	XZ-C	XZ-C	xz-c	XZ-C
gastric cancer	ascites					
	cancer cell					

XZ-C4+5

Medical history and treatment:

On June 1, 1994, a 3cmX 3cm deep ulcer of the gastric antrum was found under a gastroscope, and the cytological examination revealed gastric cancer.

Radical gastric cancer was performed in June 1994. Cancer cells invaded the muscle layer, but no minor curvature metastasis was seen. Pathological examination revealed gastric mucinous cell adenocarcinoma.

In early May 1996, he was found to have abdominal distension, pain, anorexia, and fatigue.

On May 14, 1996, he was admitted to the Department of Traditional Chinese Medicine of Xiehe Hospital. He had fever, abdominal pain, low protein, ascites, and pleural fluid.

Ascites examination has cancer cells.

Due to full abdominal distension and uncomfortable abdominal distension, after various treatments, the ascites did not go away, so the patient was transferred to the Integrative Chinese and Western Medicine Anticancer Research Collaborative Group XZ-C series of immunological Chinese medicine treatment.

After taking XZ-C series of immune-regulating and control Chinese medicines, the patient's appetite was improved.

The ascites was from gradually subsided to completely subsided, and the physical strength was obviously improved.

The patient came to the clinic every month for rechecks and took XZ-C medicine.

In June 1996, the patient came to the clinic with the XZ-C series of more immunological regulation and control Chinese medicine treatments.

It has been 6 years after gastric cancer surgery, and 4 years have passed since recurrence and metastasis.

As of December 1999, the patient was generally in good condition, with good mental appetite, and his appearance was healthy and normal. See the above figure.

Evaluation:

This patient had gastric cancer surgery in June 1994, and no other treatment was given after the operation (due to chemotherapy response). There were cancer cells in the pleural and ascites in May 1996. Because of the severe ascites, he did not receive any radiotherapy or chemotherapy. He insisted on taking XZ-C. With a series of immune regulation and control Chinese medicine, the patient has recovered well, and it has been 4 years since the follow-up visit, and his health is good.

This example prompts:

One year after gastric cancer, there are cancer cells in the pleural fluid and ascites, which recur and metastasize.

The XZ-C1+4 immunomodulatory Chinese medicine controls the tumor cells, so that the pleural fluid and ascites subsides, the condition improves, and the patient's health is restored, which means that XZ-C1+4 can help with controlling pleural effusion and ascites cancer; control recurrence and metastasis of cancer and it improves the quality of life and the patient lives longer with tumors.

Case 19

Wang XXX, male, 53 years old farmer Xinzhou
Medical record number: xxxx

Diagnosis:

anastomotic recurrence after gastric cancer

The figure of diagnosis and treatment of anastomotic recurrence after gastric cancer surgery is as the following:

1994.06	1994.7	1994.8	1995.5. 30	1996. 6.2	1996	1997
Surgery	Chemotherapy	Chemotherapy	GI recurrence	XZ-C	XZ-C	XZ-C

XZ-C1+4+2

Medical history and treatment:

The patient began to feel retrosternal discomfort in February 1994.

In May 1994, the local hospital confirmed gastric cancer by gastroscopy.

178

At the end of June 1994, he was given a radical resection of gastric cancer, followed by 2 courses of postoperative chemotherapy with 5-Fu+MMC.

On May 30, 1995, the Tongji Hospital re-examined. After a barium meal, it was found that the anastomotic mucosa was damaged, about 5cm long, and the anastomotic stoma was obviously narrow and not smooth. It was a recurrence of the anastomotic stoma. A local area with a diameter of about 5cm was visible.

The patient started to take XZ-C1+4 immune-regulating Chinese medicine for a long time at the cooperative anti-cancer clinic on June 2, 1995.

After taking the medicine, my general condition improved, my appetite was good, the patient could eat dry rice or steamed buns, and had better eating significantly improved compared with before, and it had been 2 and a half years at the time of follow-up, and the condition was good. See the above figure.

Evaluation:

This case was a recurrence of anastomotic cancer after gastric cancer, and the anastomotic stenosis could not be operated on. He started taking XZ-C anti-cancer immune Chinese medicine in June 1995. It has been 2 and a half years since the follow-up visit and the condition is good.

This example prompts:

XZ-C immunomodulatory Chinese medicine can stabilize recurrent cancer without developing, and get better, and the symptoms will be significantly improved.

Long-term survival with tumors means that XZ-C1+4 can achieve better results when used for recurrent cancer.

Case 20

Zhang xxx, Female, 39 years old, Accountant from Wuhan
Medical record number: xxxx

Diagnosis:

cancerous gastric ulcer, poorly differentiated adenocarcinoma

The figure of diagnosis and treatment of poorly differentiated gastric adenocarcinoma is as the following:

1994.4.20		1995.11.22	1996	1997	1998	1999	2000	2005
Surgery	Postoperative Chemotherapy 6 times	XZ-C	XZ-C	XZ-C	XZ-C	XZ-C	XZ-C	XZ-C

XZ-Cl+4+5

Medical history and treatment:

In March 1994, due to epigastric discomfort for 1 month and worsening for 1 week, gastroscope showed gastric ulcer.

On April 20, 1994, he underwent a subtotal gastrectomy, 6 postoperative chemotherapy (5-FU+MMC) and liver protection treatment, and the pathological section after the operation showed poorly differentiated gastric cancer with lymph node metastasis.

On November 22, 1995, he came to the outpatient clinic of the Anti-cancer Research Cooperation Group of Integrated Traditional Chinese and Western Medicine to use XZ-Cl+4+5 immunomodulatory anti-cancer Chinese medicine. No other treatments were used.

Long-term medication was used to promote the immune function and to have the protection of the bone marrow. By the time of return, it was more than 10 years, no recurrence or metastasis occurred, and the condition was good. See the above figure.

Analysis and evaluation:

This patient has a poorly differentiated adenocarcinoma of the stomach with lymph node metastasis.

Subtotal gastrectomy was performed on April 20, 1994, and chemotherapy was performed 6 times after surgery.

From November 22, 1995, XZ-Cl+4+8 immunomodulatory Chinese medicine was used only, and no other drugs were used for treatment. It has been 10 years and it is in good condition.

This example prompts:

Postoperative chemotherapy plus long-term use of XZ-C immuno-regulatory anticancer medicine can improve the long-term effect. After surgery, supplemented with XZ-C immuno-regulatory and control anti-cancer medicine can prevent postoperative recurrence and metastasis.

Case 21

Zhou XXX, male, 57 years old, Huanggang cadre
Medical record number: xxxx

Diagnosis:

Malignant transformation of gastric antrum and greater curvature ulcer

The Figure of Diagnosis and treatment of malignant transformation of gastric antrum and big bay side ulcer is as the following:

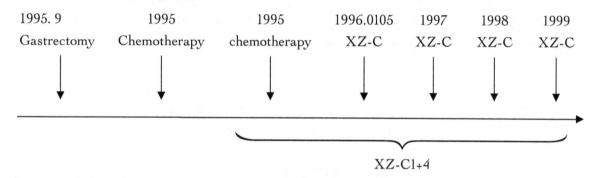

Medical history and treatment:

In September 1995, he had undergone radical resection in a local hospital for gastric cancer. After the operation, he had received 2 courses of chemotherapy.

The reaction was severe, the hair fell out and thinned.

The gastrectomy specimen was moderately differentiated adenocarcinoma, and no lymphatic metastasis was found in the omentum.

The patient came to the outpatient clinic of the Anti-cancer Research Cooperation Group of Integrated Traditional Chinese and Western Medicine on January 5, 1996, and treated with XZ-C1+4.

The general condition improved, and the spirit and appetite were good. Long-term use of XZ-C immune traditional Chinese medicine is to protect Thymus and increase immune function, and the patient has been on the XZ-C medication for 4 years and is in good condition. See the above picture.

Evaluation:

This case was malignant gastric ulcer and moderately differentiated adenocarcinoma.

It was radically resectioned on September 25, 1995. Two courses of chemotherapy were given in February after the operation.

The response was large and it was not done again. It was only treated with XZ-C immunoregulatory Chinese medicine in order to prevent recurrence and metastasis, it has been 4 years and in good condition by the time of follow-up visit.

This case suggests that due to the significant decline in immune function after gastric cancer surgery, short-term chemotherapy plus long-term long-term XZ-Cl+4 immunoregulatory Chinese medicine after gastric surgery can protect Thymus and increase immune function, and improve the overall immune function, and prevent recurrence and metastasis of gastric cancer.

Case 22

Yin xxx, Male 58 years old from Shanxi
Medical record number: 8801750

Diagnosis:

Postoperative gastric cancer

The Figure of Diagnosis and treatment of gastric cancer after surgery is as the following:

2000	Chemotherapy	2000.	2001	2002	2003	2004	2005	2006	2007	2008	2009	2010
4.27	Once	6.19	XZ-C	XZ-C	XZ-C	XZ-C	XZ-C	XZ-C	XZ-C	XZ-C	XZ-C	XZ-C
Radical		XZ-C										
Surgery												
for Gastric												
Cancer												

Serve XZ-Cl+4

Medical history and treatment:

Stomach pain for two years, gastric cancer was diagnosed by gastroscopy.

Radical gastric cancer surgery was performed in Union Hospital on April 27, 2000. Postoperative pathology: poorly differentiated adenocarcinoma of the gastric body.

The patient had chemotherapy for 5 days after surgery.

On June 19, 2000, the patient came to Shuguang Cancer Specialist Clinic to use XZ-C immunomodulatory Chinese medicine for postoperative adjuvant treatment, and **used XZ-C1+4 to protect the Thymus and promote immunity. The pa**tient insisted on taking the medicine for a long time to enhance immunity. It has been 11 years. She was in good health when she came to the clinic for follow-up on January 8, 2010. See the above figure.

Analysis and evaluation:

This patient received chemotherapy after radical surgery for gastric cancer, but because of the high response, he continued to take XZ-C immune-regulating and control anti-cancer Chinese medicine to protect Thymus and increase, and protect bone marrow and promote the production of blood, improve the body's anti-cancer immunity and prevent recurrence, transfer, the patient has been insisting on taking a small amount of medicine, and has been in good health for 11 years.

Case 23

Zeng XXX, female, 54 years old, worker
Medical record number: xxxx

Diagnosis:

Gastric Adenocarcinoma

The Figure of Diagnosis and treatment of gastric adenocarcinoma is as the following:

2002. 10.14 Radical Surgery	Chemotherapy once	2002. 10.25	2003	2004	2005	2006	2007	2008	2009	2010
		XZ-C	XZ-C	XZ-C	XZ-C	XZ-C	XZ-C	XZ-C	XZ-C	XZ-C

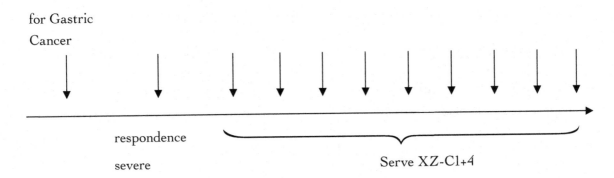

for Gastric
Cancer

respondence

severe

Serve XZ-Cl+4

Medical history and treatment:

Gastroscopy in September 2002 was gastric cancer. Radical gastric cancer surgery was performed in Wuhan Third Hospital on October 14, 2002.

Postoperative pathology: gastric adenocarcinoma I-II, infiltrating deep muscle layer, lymph node metastasis 2/3, postoperative chemotherapy once, WBC decreased so that chemotherapy was stopped.

On October 25, 2002, Mi Shuguang Cancer Specialist Clinic used XZ-Cl+4 immunomodulation for postoperative and adjuvant treatment. After taking the medicine, the spirit and appetite were good, and the physical strength gradually recovered. It has been 8 years since the medicine has been taken.

On the 4th of September 2010 when the patient came to the outpatient clinic for follow-up visits, his health recovered well. See the above Figure.

Analysis and evaluation:

This patient received chemotherapy after surgery for gastric cancer, but the response was big, but he did not do it again. Instead, he came to the outpatient clinic to take XZ-C immunoregulatory traditional Chinese medicine, which is an adjuvant treatment after surgery to protect the Thymus and increase immune function; protect bone marrow and promote the production of blood, improve immunity and prevent recurrence and metastasis, the patient insisted on long-term small-dose medication for 8 years, and has good health.

Case 24

Ni XXX, male, 60 years old, Wuhan Jiangxia, Medical record number: xxxx

Diagnosis:

Stomach Antral Cancer

The figure of Diagnosis and treatment of gastric antrum cancer is as the following:

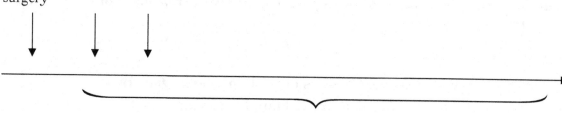

1998,12	1999. 1. 31	2000	2001	2002	2003	2004	2005	2006	2007	2008	2009	2010
Stomach cancer surgery	XZ-C	XZ-C	XZ-C	XZ-C	XZ-C	XZ-C	XZ-C	XZ-C	XZ-C	XZ-C	XZ-C	XZ-C

Serve XZ-C1+4.

Medical history and treatment:

The patient had pain under the area of back heart and xiphoid process for 4 months.

After gastroscopy and biopsy, it was a poorly differentiated adenocarcinoma of the gastric antrum.

Radical subtotal gastrectomy was performed in Xiehe Hospital in December 1998. The postoperative pathology was the same as above, with metastasis to lesser curved lymph nodes (2/6) and metastasis to greater curved lymph nodes (1/8).

No chemotherapy was given after the operation.

The patient came to Shuguang Oncology Clinic on January 31, 1999 for postoperative adjuvant treatment of integrated traditional Chinese and Western medicine.

Taking XZ-C1+4, after taking the medicine, the mental appetite is good, the physical strength is restored, and the long-term use of XZ-C regulating traditional Chinese medicine is adhered to, and the outpatient visits and medicine are taken once a month. It has been 12 years and the health condition is good. See the above picture.

Analysis and evaluation:

This patient received radical surgery for gastric cancer without chemotherapy, and came to the clinic one month after the operation.

Immune regulation and control therapy was used to protect Thymus and increase the immune function, protect bone marrow and to produce blood, prevent recurrence and metastasis, and insist on long-term small-dose medication. It has been 12 years and is in good health.

Fourth, some typical cases of postoperative adjuvant treatment of lung cancer

Case 25

Di * *, Male, 68 years old, Changzhou, Qian Bu
Medical record number: xxxx

Diagnosis:

Central lung cancer of the right upper lung with metastasis to the left lung

The figure of diagnosis and treatment of lung cancer cases is as the following:

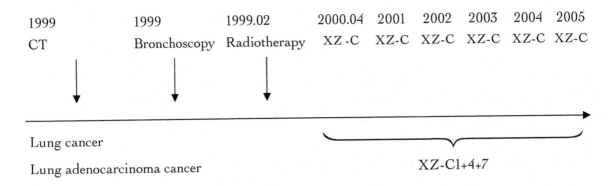

1999	1999	1999.02	2000.04	2001	2002	2003	2004	2005
CT	Bronchoscopy	Radiotherapy	XZ-C	XZ-C	XZ-C	XZ-C	XZ-C	XZ-C

Lung cancer

Lung adenocarcinoma cancer   XZ-C1+4+7

Medical history and treatment:

He coughed for 2 weeks in October 1998, accompanied by pain in the right shoulder, treated according to inflammation.

As of January 1999, the cough worsened, anorexia, fatigue, and weight loss. CT scan showed a mass in the upper right hilar area, which was central lung cancer.

In the Second Affiliated Hospital of Hubei Medical College, the pathological report of fiberoptic bronchoscopy and biopsy was lung adenocarcinoma.

Neither the patient nor his family agreed with the operation.

The patient received a course of radiotherapy in February 1999. The side effects were severe and the patient could not adhere to the radiotherapy. At this time, the re-examination revealed 2 lesions in the left lung, metastasis to the left lung, coughing and sputum, blood in the sputum, and shortness of breath when walking.

The patient came to Shuguang Oncology Clinic on April 23, 2000 with xz-C immunomodulation anti-cancer Chinese medicine treatment.

After taking XZ-C1+XZ-C4+XZ-C7, LMS+MDZ, after 3 months of taking the medicine, the symptoms improved. The spirit and appetite improved.

As of December 2000, the condition was stable, the spirit and appetite were good, the breathing was smooth, the complexion was ruddy, and the walking activities were normal, sometimes with a dry cough.

The patient has persisted in taking XZ-C1+4+7 daily for a long time, without interruption for more than 4 years, and has been in good health for 5 years at the time of the follow-up visit. The walking activities are like normal healthy elderly. The onset and treatment process are shown in the above figure.

Analysis and evaluation:

This patient has central lung cancer in the upper right lung.

In April 2000, The patient came to the specialist outpatient department to use XZ-C1+4+7 immunomodulatory treatment.

XZ-C1 can kill cancer red blood cells, but not normal cells;

XZ-C4 can protect Thymus and increase immune function; promotes thymic hyperplasia and improves immunity,protect bone marrow and produce blood; XZ-C7 inhibits lung cancer cells, protects lung function, and reduces phlegm and relieves cough.

Short-term radiotherapy is followed by long-term administration of xz-c immunomodulatory drugs to consolidate and enhance long-term efficacy.

The xz-c immunomodulatory drug improves the overall immune function, improves the spirit, appetite, and sleep well, helps the body's disease resistance and organ function, and restores nutrition and metabolism, which is beneficial to the recovery of the patient's health.

This patient did not undergo surgery, and received radiotherapy in February 1999. After the radiotherapy, he developed left lung metastasis. In the specialist clinic, he took XZ-C immunoregulatory anti-cancer and anti-metastasis Chinese medicine for a long time, and insisted on taking XZ-C daily for more than 4 years, without interruption, satisfactory results have been achieved, and his health has recovered well without any symptoms.

It has been 7 years since the follow-up visit.

The patient came to the outpatient clinic for follow-up visit in May 2005. The general condition is good, the spirit and appetite are good, there are no symptoms, walking, activities, talking and laughing like normal healthy elderly.

Case 26

Zhou xxx, Male, 49-year-old, Wuhan, cadre
Medical record number: xxxx

Diagnosis:

Right lower lobe lung cancer

The figure of diagnosis and treatment of lung cancer in the lower right lobe is as the following:

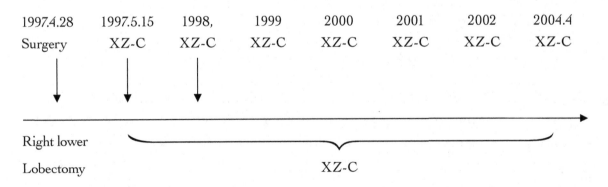

Medical history and treatment:

In 1996, chest tightness, cough, low-grade fever, and dyspnea were treated as "cold" treatment.

Sudden hemoptysis in mid-April 1997, confirmed by chest X-ray and CT examination as right lower lobe lung cancer, resection of right lower lobe lung cancer was performed in Union Hospital on April 28, 1997.

Pathology: poorly differentiated adenocarcinoma of lung.

The postoperative recovery was good. No radiotherapy or chemotherapy was done after surgery.

On May 15, 1997, I came to Shuguang Oncology Specialty Clinic to take xz-C immune regulation and control anticancer No. 1, No. 4, No. 7, vitamin C, vitamin B6, vitamin E, and vitamin A.

After taking the medicine, the general condition is good, the spirit is good, the appetite is good, the complexion is ruddy, and there is no discomfort. After taking the medicine for 3 and a half years, the condition is good, the condition is stable and controlled without recurrence or metastasis.

In June 2004, the patient came to the outpatient clinic and reported that after taking the XZ-C immunomodulatory anti-cancer drug for 3 and a half years constantly, the condition is stable. It has been 8 years and the general condition is very good, just like a healthy person. See the above Figure.

Analysis and evaluation:

This case is a poorly differentiated adenocarcinoma of the right lower lobe.

After surgical resection, there was no radiotherapy or chemotherapy. After the operation, he came to the outpatient department of Shuguang Cancer Specialist of the Integrated Traditional Chinese and Western Medicine Anti-cancer Cooperation Group to use XZ-C immunoregulatory Chinese medicine for postoperative adjuvant treatment.

After taking XZ-C1+4+7 continuously for a long time, the patient's condition recovered well, 8 years after the operation, the spirit and appetite were good, and the health condition was good.

Case 27

Zhang XXX, male, 52 years old, from Wuhan driver
Medical record number: XXXX

Diagnosis:

Right lung poorly differentiated adenocarcinoma, lymph node metastasis

The figure of diagnosis and treatment of poorly differentiated adenocarcinoma of the right lung is as the following:

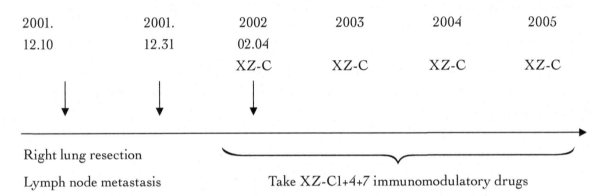

Medical history and treatment:

Due to cough and hemoptysis, CT examination showed a tumor of the right lower lung, and there was no abnormality in bronchoscopy.

On December 10, 2001, a thoracotomy was performed at the Provincial Tumor Hospital to perform a resection of the right middle and lower lobes of the right lung. During the operation, 1 lymph node in the interlobular group and 2 lymph nodes in the hilar group were seen. The pathological section of the lung was poorly differentiated adenocarcinoma. The lymph node is metastatic adenocarcinoma, and chemotherapy is given once after surgery.

The patient came to Shuguang Oncology Clinic to take XZ-C immunoregulatory anti-cancer and anti-metastasis Chinese medicine treatment on February 4, 2002.

After taking the medicine, the general condition is good, the appetite is good, and the patient insisted on taking XZ-C1+4+7, LMS, MDZ daily for 3 years, the health condition has recovered well. See the above Figure.

Analysis and evaluation:

This case is a poorly differentiated adenocarcinoma of the right lower lobe with hilar lymph node metastasis.

Postoperative chemotherapy was performed once, meanwhile, XZ-C immunomodulator XZ-C1+XZ-C4+XZ-C7 was used as postoperative adjuvant treatment.

XZ-C1 kills cancer cells but not normal cells,

XZ-C4 protects the thymus, improves immunity, protects the marrow and promote the production of blood;

XZ-C7 protects lung function. The patient has taken XZ-C immunomodulatory drugs for more than 3 consecutive years to improve overall immune function and control metastasis. No distant metastasis was found. It has been 4 years at the time of follow-up. The patient is in good condition, good appetite, and walking and cctivities are as the normal healthy person.

Case 28

Long Mou, male, 60 years old, Huanggang, cadre
Medical record number XXXX.

Diagnosis:

Right middle and lower lung adenocarcinoma with mediastinal lymph node metastasis.

The figure of diagnosis and treatment of right middle and lower lung adenocarcinoma with mediastinal lymph node metastasis is as the following:

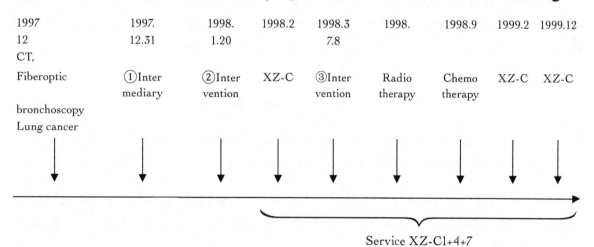

Medical history and treatment:

Since January 1997, he often coughed and fever, and was treated as pneumonia.

CT showed cancer of the lower right lung in December 1997. Fiberoptic bronchoscopy showed that the right lower central type poorly differentiated adenocarcinoma with mediastinal lymphatic metastasis The patient was treated with intervention + XZ-C Chinese medicine.

The first bronchial artery intervention was done on December 31, 1997.

The second intervention on January 20, 1998,

The third intervention in March 1998,

35 times of radiotherapy were done on July 8, 1998.

After the radiotherapy ended in September 1998, another 2 courses (1 month) of chemotherapy were given.

From February 14 to March 14, 1998, from May 9 to June 9, and from July 1 to August 1, the patient took XZ-C1 + XZ-C4+ XZ-C7 immune traditional Chinese medicine, the cough decreased, general condition is good, mental appetite is good, physical strength is restored, walking activities as usual, dry cough without sputum after taking the medicine.

On August 9, 1998, the patient developed radiation esophagitis, mucosal edema, congestion, dysphagia, and hoarseness were caused by radiotherapy. The patient started to take XZ-C Chinese medicine atomization to inhale. Radiation pneumonia and pleural effusion occurred again. The patient continues taking the XZ-C series of medicines, after taking these medications, the spirit and appetite improved and the patient can eat without discomfort. See the above picture.

Analysis and evaluation:

In this case, mediastinal lymphatic metastasis of the lower right lung cancer was treated with intervention + XZ-C Chinese medicine.

Long-term administration of XZ-C immune regulation and control Chinese medicine was done. The general condition is good, and the appetite is good. It has been 2 years and 8 months at the time of follow-up.

This case prompts:

The lower left lung cancer has metastasis to the mediastinum and cannot be operated. It is treated with intermediary + radiotherapy + Chinese medicine. Radiotherapy + intermediary chemotherapy is used to kill the cancerous cancer cells, followed by XZ-C immunoregulatory Chinese medicine to protect Thymus and increase the immune function, and to improve the body's overall immune level and to consolidate the curative effect and prevent recurrence, and achieved good results.

Case 29

Xie, male, 55 years old, Xiangfan, medical record number xxxx.

Diagnosis:

Adenocarcinoma of the upper right lung.

The Figure of Diagnosis and treatment of right upper lung adenocarcinoma is as the following:

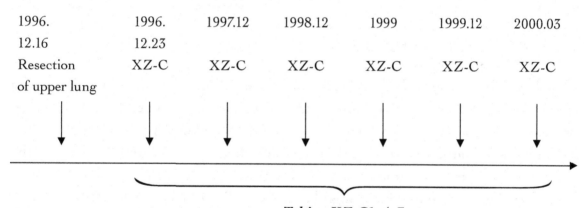

1996.12.16	1996.12.23	1997.12	1998.12	1999	1999.12	2000.03
Resection of upper lung	XZ-C	XZ-C	XZ-C	XZ-C	XZ-C	XZ-C

Taking XZ-Cl+4+7

Medical history and treatment:

The power of the right shoulder and right hand was weakened for half a year, and he coughed 2 months ago, with little sputum and no blood sputum.

On November 26, 1996, chest x-ray film of the upper right lung spherical lesion.

CT diagnosis was confirmed as upper right lung cancer on December 4, 1996.

The upper right lung lobectomy was performed on December 16, 1996, and the pathological report was adenocarcinoma of the right upper lung.

On December 23, 1996, he came to the outpatient clinic of the Anti-cancer Cooperation Group of Integrated Chinese and Western Medicine to take XZ-C Chinese medicine to prevent recurrence and metastasis. No other treatment was used after the operation.

He has been taking XZ-C medicine for a long time, and he is generally in good condition, with good mental appetite, good physical recovery, and no symptoms. The complexion is ruddy, it has been 3 and a half years, everything is good, like a healthy person. In the past 2 years, multiple chest X-ray examinations showed changes after lung surgery, and no abnormalities were changed. There were no abnormalities in liver B-ultrasound. See the above Figure.

Analysis and evaluation:

This case has been treated with XZ-C1 +XZ-C4 +XZ-C7 for 3 and a half years after surgery, and is still taking XZ-C immune regulation and control Chinese medicine, without radiotherapy and chemotherapy, and is in good health, just like a normal healthy person.

The Tip of this case is as the following

After lung cancer surgery, taking XZ-C immunomodulatory Chinese medicine for a longer period of time can be regulated and controlled for a longer period of time to prevent recurrence and metastasis. Because XZ-C medicine protects Thymus and increase the immune function, and protects the bone marrow and to promote the production of blood, and improves the overall immune function, the patient's immune ability has been maintained at a high level. No radiotherapy or chemotherapy was used after the operation, and the XZ-C immune control Chinese medicine was used alone. He is in good condition and is as strong as a normal healthy person.

This example prompts:

After lung cancer surgery, the patient takes XZ-C immunomodulatory Chinese medicine for a longer period of time, which can be adjusted for a longer period of time to prevent recurrence and metastasis.

Because XZ-C medicine protects Thymus and increases immune function, and protects the marrow and to promote the production of blood, and improves the overall immune function, the patient's immune function has been maintained at a high level. No radiotherapy or chemotherapy was used after the operation. The XZ-C immune control and regulation Chinese medicine was only used. He is in good condition and is as strong as a normal healthy person.

Case 30

Huang Mou, male, 54 years old, Xiaogan, cadre
Medical record number xxxx.

Diagnosis:

The lung squamous cell carcinoma of left low lobe

The figure of diagnosis and treatment of lung squamous cell carcinoma of left low lobe is as the following:

1997. 8.31	1997. 9.19	1998.9	1999.4	2000.3
Lower left lung resection	XZ-C	XZ-C	XZ-C	XZ-C

Taking XZ-C1+4+7, and the health is restored

Medical history and treatment:

In September 1996, he coughed up sputum with blood, and improved according to inflammation treatment.

He had hemoptysis again in April 1997. The local treatment could not stop the blood.

It was diagnosed as squamous cell carcinoma by a tissue biopsy on August 15, 1997 with fiberoptic bronchoscopy + bronchography.

The left lower lobectomy was performed at Union Hospital on August 31, 1997, and the disease was found to be left lower lung squamous cell carcinoma with hilar lymph node metastasis (1/3).

On September 19, 1997, he came to the collaborative group for treatment with XZ-C immune regulation and control traditional Chinese medicine to prevent recurrence and metastasis.

After taking the medicine, the spirit and appetite are good, and the general condition is good. I will come to the clinic every month for review and take XZ-C immune regulation Chinese medicine.

The patient came to the clinic for review in April 1999.

The general condition is good, the complexion is ruddy, walking, activities, talking and laughing are normal, the neck is supraclavicular (0), both underarms (0), liver and spleen (0), weight 63kg, chest x-ray film and the CT report was a postoperative change.

After the operation, he came to the clinic to take XZ-C1 + XZ-C2 + XZ-C7 for two and a half years. He has not been treated with radiotherapy, chemotherapy or other methods, and his health has recovered well. See the above picture.

Analysis and evaluation:

This case underwent a left lower lobectomy on August 31, 1997. The disease was examined as left lower lung squamous cell carcinoma with hilar lymph node metastasis (1/3). He came to the outpatient clinic of the Chinese and Western Medicine Anti-cancer Cooperation Group on September 19, 1997 for treating with XZ-C1 + XZ-C4 +XZ-C7 immunomodulatory Chinese medicine, and the patient has no other radiotherapy or chemotherapy, has been nearly 3 years, and the health condition has recovered well.

This case suggests that after lung cancer resection, the use of XZ-C1 +XZ-C4 +XZ-C7 immunoregulatory Chinese medicine can improve the immune function and enhance physical situation, maintain the therapeutic effect, make the body form an in vivo environment that is not conducive to the proliferation of cancer cells, thereby preventing cancer recurrence.

Case 31

Wang, male, 61 years old, Macheng, cadre.

Diagnosis:

Left lung central lung cancer.

The figure of diagnosis and treatment of left lung central lung cancer is as the following:

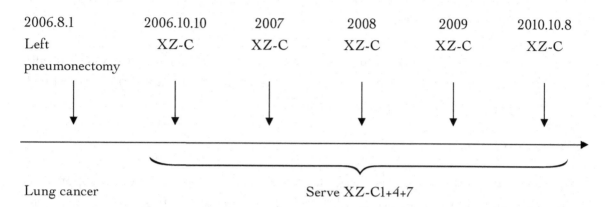

2006.8.1	2006.10.10	2007	2008	2009	2010.10.8
Left pneumonectomy	XZ-C	XZ-C	XZ-C	XZ-C	XZ-C

Lung cancer   Serve XZ-Cl+4+7

Medical history and treatment:

On July 29, 2006, a physical examination revealed a tumor in the left lung.

On August 21, 2006, he received an intrapericardial pneumonectomy, mediastinal lymph node removal, partial pericardial resection + partial left atrial resection + lunar broom nerve transection at Tongji Hospital. The operation went smoothly. The left pneumothorax was recovered 7 days after the operation, and it recovered after drainage.

After the operation, due to frailty, radiotherapy and chemotherapy were not performed.

The patient came to Shuguang Oncology Clinic on October 10, 2006 to take XZ-Cl+4+7 immune regulation and control medication as the postoperative adjuvant treatment. After taking the medicine, the spirit and appetite are good, and the physical strength is gradually restored. The patient is adhere to long-term medication and comes every month. It has been 5 years for outpatient follow-up visits and medicine collection.

He came to the clinic for medicine on October 8, 2010, and was in good health. See the above figure.

Analysis and evaluation:

In this case, the central type of left lung cancer was difficult to operate. Pneumonectomy in the pericardium + mediastinal lymph node dissection + partial pericardiotomy + partial left atrial resection of the ten septum was performed.

After the operation, the left pneumothorax was re-drained and recovered.

No radiotherapy or chemotherapy was allowed afterwards.

The patient came to Shuguang Oncology Clinic to take xz-C1 +4 +7 immunomodulation therapy on November 11, 2006.

The patient is adhere to long-term medication, and return to the clinic every month to get the medicine. He has recovered well, with good spirits and good appetite. It has been 5 years and he is in good health.

This case prompts:

Central left lung lung cancer is difficult to surgically remove. After the operation, the immune function is low and the physical strength is weak. It is more appropriate to use XZ-C immunoregulatory Chinese medicine for postoperative adjuvant treatment. It is more appropriate to protect Thymus and increase immune function, and to promote the production of blood. This patient is recovering well.

Case 32

Guan Mou, male, 64 years old, Foshan, Guangdong, entrepreneur, Medical record number XXXX

Diagnosis:

Right lung adenocarcinoma.

The Figure of Diagnosis and treatment of right lung adenocarcinoma is as the following:

2005.5.16	2005.5	2005 7.13	2006	2007	2008	2009	2010
Right	Chemotherapy once	XZ-C	XZ-C	XZ-C	XZ-C	XZ-C	XZ-C

Lung
Upper
lobectomy

peripheral

lung cancer

Serve XZ-C1+4+7+LMS+MDZ

Medical history and treatment:

In May 2005, CT in Nanfang Hospital found peripheral lung cancer of the right lung.

On May 16, 2005, the right upper lobectomy was performed at the Fifth Hospital of Foshan City.

Postoperative pathology:

(upper right lung) peripheral lung adenocarcinoma, alveolar and papillary differentiation, no cancer in the lymph nodes.

The patient had postoperative chemotherapy once, came to Shuguang Oncology Clinic on July 13, 2005 for XZ-C immunoregulation Traditional Chinese medicine as an adjuvant treatment for lung cancer after surgery.

After taking XZ-C1 + XZ-C4 + XZ-C7 + LMS + MDZ, the general condition is good, the appetite is good, and the recovery is good.

After the operation, the patient simply took the above-mentioned XZ-C1 +XZ-C, +XZ-C7 immune-regulating and control Chinese medicine without other treatments, and took XZ-C1 +XZ-C4 +XZ-C7 +LMS+MDZ daily for more than 5 years. The patient has Good health. See the above figure.

Analysis and evaluation:

This case was a right upper lobe lung cancer undergoing a right upper lobectomy.

The postoperative chemotherapy was performed once.

The response was large and no further treatment.

He came to the specialist outpatient clinic in July 2005 to take XZ-C1 +4 +7 every 3 months. He returned to the outpatient clinic for medicine. After taking the medicine, he had a good appetite and no other treatment. He insisted on taking medicine for a long time. It has been more than 5 years and he is in good health.

Case 33

Lin, female, 64 years old, from Dalian, medical record number XXXX.

Diagnosis:

After right lung cancer surgery, both lung metastases and bone metastases.

The figure of diagnosis and treatment of lung metastases and bone metastases after right lung cancer surgery is as the following :

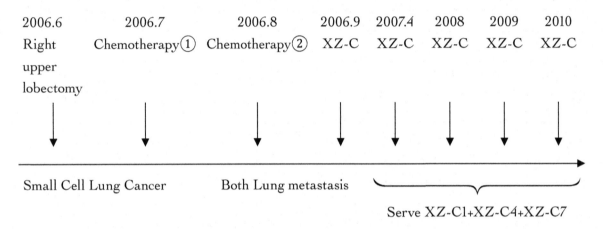

Medical history and treatment:

In March 2006, there was no cause for irritating cough;

CT in May 2006 showed lung cancer in the upper right.

He underwent right upper lobectomy + lymph node dissection in the Second Hospital of Dalian Medical University in June 2006.

The postoperative pathology was small cell lung cancer.

The patient had Postoperative chemotherapy in July 2006, CE regimen for 2 cycles, III degree of bone marrow suppression.

A re-examination of CT at 9 months after surgery showed multiple nodules in both lungs, suggesting metastases in both lungs.

Due to the purchase of the book "New Concepts and New Methods for Cancer Metastasis Treatment", on April 3, 2007 the patient came to Shuguang Cancer Specialist Clinic to use XZ-C1+XZ-C4+XZ-C7 + LMS+ Vit immunomodulation anti-cancer Chinese medicine treatment. The patient is adhere to long-term medication, more than 4 years so far, the patient is generally in good condition, good spirit and appetite, walking activities like healthy elderly. See the above picture.

Analysis and evaluation:

This case is a small cell lung cancer of the right upper lung. The postoperative chemotherapy was performed twice, and the bone marrow band was suppressed. He came to the outpatient clinic with XZ-C immunoregulatory Chinese medicine treatment, it is to protect Thymus and increase immune function, promot marrow protection, as an adjuvant treatment after surgery. I have been taking long-term medication for more than 4 years and have controlled the transfer.

This example prompts:

XZ-C immune regulation Chinese medicine can be used as an adjuvant treatment for lung cancer after surgery, which can improve the immune function of patients and prevent recurrence and metastasis.

4. **Typical cases of adjuvant treatment after esophageal cancer**

Case 34

Ding, male, 63 years old, Wuhan, cadre, medical record number XXXX.

Diagnosis:

Cancer of the middle esophagus.

The figure of diagnosis and treatment of cancer of the middle esophagus is as the following:

1994. 02.03		1995. 04.05	1996	1997	1998	1999	2000. 5	2001	2010
Radical Mastectomy	postoperative radiotherapy + immunotherapy	XZ-C	XZ-C	XZ-C	XZ-C	X Z-C	XZ -C	XZ-C	XZ-C

$\longrightarrow$

XZ-C1+4 alone, no chemotherapy, 16 years, good health

Medical history and treatment:

Progressive dysphagia occurred in January 1994 and was diagnosed by barium swallow examination.

On February 3 of the same year, he underwent radical resection of middle esophageal cancer, neck esophagus-gastric anastomosis, and 1-month postoperative radiotherapy.

Due to heart problems, there is no postoperative chemotherapy.

On April 5, 1995, the patient came to the outpatient clinic of the Combination of Chinese and Western Medicine Anti-cancer Cooperation Group, using XZ-C1+4 immunoregulatory Chinese medicine treatment, after taking the medicine, the spirit and appetite are good, and the physical strength is restored.

From 1996 to 1999, once a month the patient comes to outpatient follow-up visits and medicine collection and has long-term adherence to XZ-C1 + XZ-C4, in good condition.

At the follow-up visit in July 2005, the patient's hair was gray, and his hair has gradually become black for more than a year.

Now he has black hair, and his facial skin is softer than before, and his complexion is ruddy.

He is a completely healthy old man. It has been 16 years and he is still taking XZ-C Chinese medicine. See the above picture.

Analysis and evaluation:

This case underwent radical mastectomy for middle esophageal cancer on February 3, 1994, and received radiotherapy and immunotherapy 40 days after the operation. After that, he took XZ-C1+4 immunoregulatory Chinese medicine for a long time. It has been 16 years and he is in good health.

Treatment experience of this patient:

Radiotherapy and immunotherapy were done within 40 days after operation.

After 40 days, the patient took XZ-C1+4 immune regulation and control Chinese medicine for a long time, protect Thymus and increase immune function and promote immunity, protect the bone marrow and promote the production of blood.

XZ-C1 can inhibit cancerous cells, and XZ-C4 can promote immunity, induce cancer suppressor factors, improve the overall immune system function, protect immune organs, and eliminate the recurrence factors of dormant cells entering the proliferation stage.

Long-term continuous medication keeps the body at a high level of immune function for a long time, prevents recurrence and metastasis, and restores health.

Case 35

Huang, female, 66 years old, Wuhan Hanyang, medical record number xxxx

Diagnosis:

Poorly differentiated squamous cell carcinoma of the lower esophagus.

The Figure of Diagnosis and treatment of esophageal cancer cases is as the following :

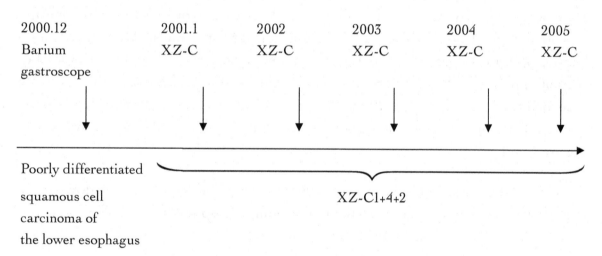

Medical history and treatment:

In December 2000, the patient was vomiting, progressive dysphagia, obstruction of eating, only half-liquid food and on esophageal gastroscopy it was showing that there was lower esophageal stenosis, congestion, erosion, small ulcers and **biopsy pathology report of poorly differentiated squamous cell carcinoma of the lower esophagus.**

Surgical treatment should be considered according to the condition, but due to financial difficulties, surgery is not possible, so the patient came to Shuguang Cancer Specialty Clinic to use XZ-C immunoregulatory anti-cancer medicine XZ-C1+XZ-C4+XZ-C2 for integrated Chinese and Western medicine treatment.

After taking the medicine for 1 month, the spirit and appetite improved, and the patient himself had better eating, and he could take vermicelli and porridge. The patient continues to take XZ-C1 + XZ-C4 + XZ-C2 for 6 months, and have a good spirit and appetite. The patient can eat soft rice, noodles, and porridge.

He continued to take XZ-C immunomodulatory anti-cancer Chinese medicine XZ-C1+4+2.

By June 2003, the patient had been taking XZ-C medicine for 2 and a half years.

The general condition and mental appetite were acceptable, and he could eat ordinary rice. There is no discomfort, eat like normal people.

The drug was stopped for 4 and a half months. After eating fried noodle nests and fried dough sticks on October 16, 2003, it suddenly caused obstruction and vomiting of coffee-colored liquid. The patient could not eat for 3 days. After rehydration support therapy improved, the patient continued to take XZ-C1+4 + 2 until October 31, 2003, he was able to take general food again, and he did not stop the drug. He returned to the clinic in May 2005. Now he is in his 70s and is like a healthy elderly person. The general condition is good, the appetite is good, and he can always take general food.

There is no discomfort and the patient is living on the 7th floor and can go downstairs every day, and sometimes can do the job of pumping up the bicycle. The onset and treatment process are shown in the above Figure.

Analysis and evaluation:

This patient was a poorly differentiated squamous cell carcinoma of the lower esophagus. It was confirmed by gastroscopy and biopsy pathology.

He could only take liquid and a small amount of semi-liquid food when he came to the clinic. The patient relied on the bicycle to maintain his life.

Due to financial difficulties, he could not undergo surgery or radiotherapy, or chemotherapy.

After taking XZ-C immunomodulatory Chinese medicine for a long time without other treatment, the symptoms improved significantly after taking the medicine for half a year.

After taking the medicine for 2 and a half years, he completely recovered as a normal healthy person. There was no discomfort after taking the general meal. He was ordered to do a barium meal review, but he was unwilling to do it due to economic reasons. In recent years, eating and living are as uncomfortable as normal healthy people. It has been 5 years since the follow-up visit and the condition is good.

Long-term use of XZ-C immune regulation anti-cancer Chinese medicine can improve the patient's immunity and improve the patient's spirit and sleep.

XZ-C4 can protect the marrow and promote the production of blood, protect Thymus and promote immunity, promote the improvement of nutrition and metabolism, **remove free radicals**, and is beneficial to the control and repair of lesions.

Case 36

Huang, female, 65 years old, Hubei Huangpo, farmer, medical record number xxxx.

Diagnosis:

Cancer of the middle esophagus.

The Figure of Diagnosis and treatment of middle esophageal cancer is as the following:

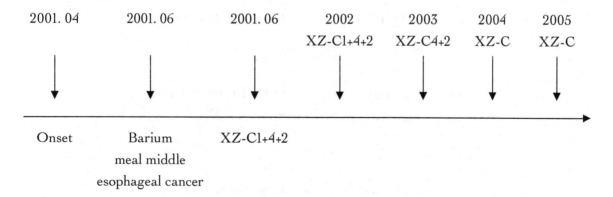

Medical history and treatment conditions:

Swallowing obstruction began in April 2001, chest and back pain and discomfort, gradually worsening, and by June, he could only consume liquid food and spit sputum.

On June 6, 2001, a barium examination at Xiehe Hospital showed a stenosis of about 10cm in length 2cm under the aortic arch.

A shallow arc-shaped filling defect of about 6cm in length was seen on the left wall, and the membrane was interrupted and damaged. Because of financial difficulties, he was unable to undergo surgery, radiotherapy, and chemotherapy.

On June 25, 2001, he came to the Shuguang Oncology Clinic to take the XZ-C immune-regulating and control anti-cancer medicine XZ-C1+4 +2 treatment. After taking the medicine for 3 months, the patient's general condition is good, the appetite is good, and the difficulty in swallowing gradually improves. The patient can eat rice porridge and noodles. The patient continued to take XZ-C1+4+2.

By March 2002, the patient can gradually eat rice and general Food.

It changed to XZ-C1+XZ-C2 in July 2003, and returned in April 2005. The patient's general condition is good, and the mental appetite is good. He has been taking XZ-C immunomodulatory drugs for 5 years and is in good condition, and the patient can eat general food, and able to do light housework. See the above Figure.

Analysis and evaluation:

This patient has middle esophageal cancer. He has not undergone surgery, radiotherapy or chemotherapy. He orally takes immunoregulatory anti-cancer medicine XZ-C1+XZ-C4+XZ-C2. He has been taking the medicine for 4 years without metastasis. He has been controlled, and the patient is recovering well. At present, the patient can eat ordinary rice without discomfort. Like other healthy elderly people, the patient can do some housework and still continue to take XZ-C4+2 Chinese medicine.

Case 37

Huang Mou, male, 66 years old, Huang Po, cadre, medical record number XXXX

Diagnosis:

Middle and lower esophagus cancer.

The Figure of Diagnosis and treatment of middle and lower esophagus cancer is as the following:

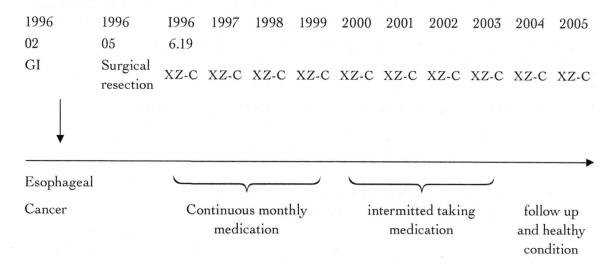

1996	1996	1996	1997	1998	1999	2000	2001	2002	2003	2004	2005
02	05	6.19									
GI	Surgical resection	XZ-C	XZ-C	XZ-C	XZ-C	XZ-C	XZ-C	XZ-C	XZ-C	XZ-C	XZ-C

Esophageal

Cancer

Continuous monthly medication   intermitted taking medication   follow up and healthy condition

Medical history and treatment:

The patient has eating obstruction in March 1996, barium in late April to diagnose cancer of the middle and lower esophagus.

Radical surgery for esophageal cancer was performed in Union Hospital in May 1996, and no other treatment was given after the operation.

On June 19, 1996, he came to the specialist outpatient clinic of the cooperative group, and used XZ-C immunomodulatory Chinese medicine as an adjuvant treatment after surgery to prevent recurrence and metastasis. The patient simply take XZ-C immune regulation Chinese medicine to protect the thymus gland to promote immunity and promote the bone marrow to produce blood.

The patient has been taking the XZ-C immune traditional Chinese medicine daily for 3 years, and later changed to intermittent use. After taking the medicine, my general condition is good, my appetite is good, and my walking activities resume as normal.

Follow-up in April 2005, the patient recovered well and often played cards in the afternoon. See the above Figure.

Analysis and evaluation:

This case did not use radiotherapy or chemotherapy after the operation of esophageal cancer, and only used XZ-C immunoregulatory Chinese medicine as an adjuvant treatment after the operation. It has been 9 years at the time of follow-up and the recovery is good.

5. **Typical cases of adjuvant treatment after breast cancer surgery**

Case 38

Chen, female, 44 years old, Wuhan, medical record number XXXX

Diagnosis:

Breast cancer.

The Figure of Diagnosis and treatment of breast cancer is as the following:

1995 2.20 Right breast cancer radical mastectomy	Postoperative radiotherapy 1 course	1995. 5.12 XZ-C	1996 XZ-C	1997 XZ-C	1998 XZ-C	1999 XZ-C	2000 XZ-C	2001 XZ-C	2002 XZ-C

Take XZ-Cl+4 continuously   Intermittent taking

Medical history and treatment:

The right breast mass was found for 3 months, and puncture biopsy was diagnosed as breast cancer.

Radical mastectomy was performed on February 20, 1995, and a course of postoperative radiotherapy was performed.

Due to poor physical strength, he could not continue, but came on May 11, 1995 Cooperative group outpatient, using XZ-Cl+4 treatment. After taking XZ-C traditional Chinese medicine for a long time for nearly 3 years, the patient has good appetite, weight gain, physical recovery, and outpatient checkup once a month. The whole body is in good condition without other treatment. See the above Figure.

Evaluation:

This patient underwent radical mastectomy on February 20, 1995, and received 1 course of postoperative radiotherapy.

Due to poor physical strength, he could not continue. He came to the collaborative group clinic on May 11, 1995 to use XZ-Cl+4 immunomodulatory Chinese medicine for treatment. After taking the medicine for more than 3 years, the patient is in good condition. No chemotherapy has been used. The patient has been in good health for 5 years.

Case 39

Pan Mou, female, 68 years old, Shenyang.

Diagnosis:

Multiple bone metastases all over the body after radical mastectomy.

The Figure of Diagnosis and treatment of bone metastases after breast cancer surgery is as the following:

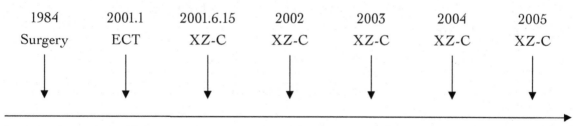

1984	2001.1	2001.6.15	2002	2003	2004	2005
Surgery	ECT	XZ-C	XZ-C	XZ-C	XZ-C	XZ-C

Bone metastasis

Medical history and treatment:

In 1984, patients with right breast cancer underwent radical mastectomy, pathological diagnosis: simple breast cancer, no lymph node metastasis.

Postoperative chemotherapy with saitepa + methotrexate has been used for 2 years, and then every year some drugs to improve the body's immunity.

In January 2001, she felt pain in his right shoulder. ECT found multiple bone metastases and enlarged right supraclavicular lymph nodes.

From March 27th, 25 radiotherapy was performed on the right supraclavicular lymph node area. During the radiotherapy, the total blood cell decreased and the white blood cell count dropped to 2.9 X 109/L. The symptoms were relieved after the radiotherapy.

On June 15, 2001, she took XZ-C immunomodulatory Chinese medicine XZ-C1+4+2, LMS, MDZ, VS. After taking the medicine for 2 months, the symptoms improved significantly. After taking the medicine for half a year, the ECT returned to normal and the condition was stable.

The patient called on September 2, 2002 and said that the physical examination was normal, especially the ECT examination returned to normal.

The patient insisted on taking the medicine every month. The patient took the XZ-C1 +XZ-C4 capsules and XZ-C2 capsules for a long time.

It has been 4 years at the time of the follow-up visit and she takes the medication without interrupted.

A call from Shenyang in April 2005 said that the patient was in good general condition, had good mental appetite, and had walking activities such as healthy elderly people. There were no abnormalities in the whole body review, liver and gallbladder ultrasound, chest X-ray film, and ECT, and the condition had recovered. See the above Figure.

Analysis and evaluation:

This case was a 17-year recurrence after radical mastectomy for right breast cancer, with extensive bone metastases throughout the body, bone destruction and pain in the right shoulder, and improved after radiotherapy.

Long-term use of XZ-C immunomodulatory Chinese medicine XZ-C1 +XZ-C4+2 has the protection of Thymus and promotes immunity, protects the bone

marrow and protects the production of blood, improves the immune function, and controls extensive bone metastasis throughout the body.

Case 40

Liu, female, 49 years old, Wuhan, accounting, medical record number XXXX45008840

Diagnosis:

Ductal carcinoma of the left breast.

The figure of the course of treatment and diagnosis of ductal carcinoma of the left breast:

1997	1997	1997.6	1997.9	1997	1998	1999	2000	2001	2002	2004
5.19	6.3			8.24						
Removal of the mass	Radical surgery	①chemo	②Chemo	XZ-C	XZ-C	XZ-C	XZ-C	XZ-C	XZ-C	XZ-C

XZ-Cl+4

Medical history and treatment:

On October 19, 1997, because the left breast mass was 3cmX3cm, the left breast mass was removed, and the section was left breast invasive ductal carcinoma.

Reoperation was performed on June 3, 1997, and radical mastectomy for left breast cancer was performed. No residual cancer was found in the residual breast tissue, and no metastasis was found in the ipsilateral axillary lymph nodes.

She received chemotherapy twice after the operation. The oral Miflon reaction was severe and did not continue.

The patient came to the outpatient clinic of the Anti-cancer Cooperation Group of Integrated Traditional Chinese and Western Medicine on August 24, 1997, and was supplemented withXZ-C immunoregulatory Chinese medicine treatment after the operation. After taking the medicine, the general condition is good, the spirit and appetite is good, and she is healthy after 3 months.

After returning to work, four months later, two masses of 3cmX3cm were found in the right breast. The boundary was unclear. The puncture cytology showed breast hyperplasia. The XZ-C1+4 Mammary Gland Hyperplasia Decoction was used, and the XZ-C immune traditional Chinese medicine was used for the past 3 years. The patient is in good condition, working as usual. See the above picture.

Analysis and evaluation:

This case was suffering from breast cancer. After radical operation, chemotherapy was performed twice. Chemotherapy was no longer used on August 24, 1997.

XZ-C immune traditional Chinese medicine alone was used as postoperative adjuvant treatment, which has Thymus protection and promotes Immune function, and marrow hemorrhage was prevented and it helps with production of blood. It can prevent from relapsing and metastasis. It has been nearly 8 years at the time of follow-up, and the condition is good.

This case suggests that

two chemotherapy treatments were used for a short period of time after breast cancer surgery. The response was large and could not be done anymore.

Later, XZ-C immunoregulatory Chinese medicine alone was used as postoperative adjuvant treatment. XZ-C1+4 can induce endogenous anti-cancer factors and induce differentiation induction, and improve the overall immune function, protect and improve the host's anti-cancer ability.

Case 41

**Li, female, 33 years old, Changde, Hunan, worker
Medical record number XXXX**

Diagnosis:

Simple cancer of the left breast.

The Figure of Diagnosis and treatment of simple breast cancer is as the following :

1996.	1996.	1996	1997	1997	1998	1999	2000	2001	2002	2003
11.29	12.25	12.29	04.02	5. 14		XZ-C	XZ-C	XZ-C	XZ-C	XZ-C
Radical	XZ-C	CMF	Chemotherapy	25 radiotherapy						
Surgery			Radiotherapy							

XZ-C1+4+ No response to radiotherapy and chemotherapy

No radiotherapy or chemotherapy was done after June 1997. It has been 6 and a half years since XZ-C medicine has been used for the follow-up visit. He is in good health. He comes to Wuchang from Changde for a follow-up visit every 3 months, such as normal people.

Medical history and treatment:

Radical mastectomy for breast cancer was performed in Changde on November 29, 1996. The right axillary lymph node metastasis (3/5), CMF chemotherapy was given one month after surgery, once a week for 4 weeks.

On December 25, 1996, the collaborative group was treated with XZ-C series drugs to protect the marrow and produce blood. After taking the medicine, the appetite is good and the blood picture rises.

From April 2, 1997 to May 14, 1997, 4 months after right breast cancer surgery + 15 times of radiotherapy on the inner side of the right breast, 15 times on the right armpit, and 25 times on the outer side of the right breast. XZ-C was used during radiotherapy. There was no reaction to radiotherapy. After taking XZ-C, the patient has been better after radiotherapy and chemotherapy, and the response is very mild, and there is basically no response.

After June 2004, the patient did not undergo radiotherapy or chemotherapy. The patient has been taking XZ-C series of medicines. The patient returns to Changde every 3 months and takes XZ-C1+4 medicines for 3 months. He persisted for a long time with good results.

He came to follow-up in December 2004. The general condition is good, the appetite is good, the complexion is ruddy, the activities are as normal, and he can do housework. The patient travels from Changde to Wuchang every three months for follow-up visits, such as healthy people. See the figure above.

Analysis and evaluation:

Treatment experience of this patient:

① Using XZ-C4 during radiotherapy and chemotherapy can alleviate the reaction, and it can be used to consolidate the long-term curative effect and prevent recurrence during the intermittent period of radiotherapy and chemotherapy.

② Six months after the operation, radiotherapy and chemotherapy + XZ-C Chinese medicine not only attack the residual cancer cells or residual small cancer foci, but also protect the host and immune organs. After six months, the general condition is good, that is, use XZ-C series to strengthen the body to eliminate evil, Consolidate the long-term effect. It has been 9 years since the operation to the follow-up visit. XZ-C immunoregulatory Chinese medicine can consolidate the long-term effect.

Case 42

**Zhang, female, 65 years old, senior engineer
Medical record number XXXX**

Diagnosis:

Ductal carcinoma of the breast

The Figure of Diagnosis and treatment of breast ductal carcinoma is as the following:

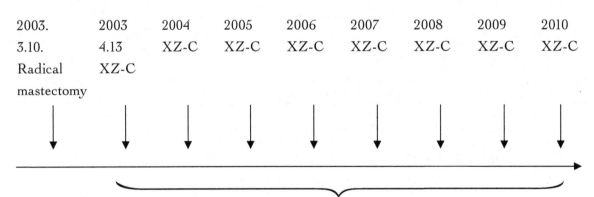

2003.	2003	2004	2005	2006	2007	2008	2009	2010
3.10.	4.13	XZ-C	XZ-C	XZ-C	XZ-C	XZ-C	XZ-C	XZ-C
Radical	XZ-C							
mastectomy								

Take XZ-C+ Shengxue Decoction

Medical history and treatment:

A physical examination at the end of 2002 revealed a small lump in the breast, which was thought to be breast cancer.

A radical mastectomy was performed at Wuhan Central Hospital on March 19, 2003.

The postoperative pathology was ductal carcinoma of the breast. No metastasis was found. He has a history of diabetes and chronic nephritis.

On April 13, 2003, he came to Shuguang Oncology Clinic to take Chinese medicine for postoperative adjuvant treatment.

He took XZ-C1+4 immunomodulatory Chinese medicine. He has been taking the medicine and visited the outpatient clinic every month. In 8 years, his health has recovered well. See the above Figure.

Analysis and evaluation:

This patient had undergone radical mastectomy. Due to chronic nephritis, he came to the specialist outpatient clinic to take XZ-C immunoregulatory anti-cancer Chinese medicine for postoperative adjuvant treatment and also took Shengxue Decoction to protect Thymus and increase immune function, protects bone marrow and products blood. Adhering to long-term medication for 8 years has not only prevented recurrence and metastasis, but the chronic nephritis has also improved significantly and has not recurred. The patient returns to the outpatient clinic for medicine every two months and is in good health.

Case 43

Liu, female, 49 years old, Changsha, Hunan, teacher, Medical record number xxxx

Diagnosis:

Infiltrating ductal carcinoma of the breast

The Figure of Diagnosis and treatment of invasive ductal carcinoma of the breast is as the following:

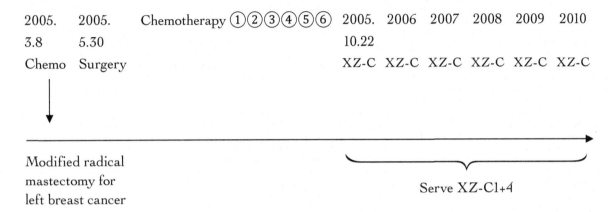

Medical history and treatment:

In February 2005, a lump in the left breast, the inner side of the left breast and a 2cmX 1.5cm nodule were found. The puncture was severely abnormal. CAF chemotherapy was performed on March 8, 2005. Partial breast resection was performed at Xiangya Hospital on May 30, 2005.

Intraoperative rapid section showed breast cancer. Retrograde modified radical mastectomy for left breast cancer. Postoperative pathology was left breast invasive ductal carcinoma, LN 0/20, immunohistochemistry C- erbB2(+ +), P53 (+), PR(-), ER(-), nm23 (+), 6 cycles of postoperative chemotherapy.

On October 22, 2005, he came to the Shuguang Oncology Clinic and took XZ-C immunoregulatory anti-cancer Chinese medicine to continue the postoperative adjuvant immunoregulation treatment to consolidate the curative effect and prevent recurrence and metastasis. See the above Figure.

Analysis and evaluation:

The patient's left axillary lymph node was preoperatively deducted, neoadjuvant chemotherapy was preoperatively followed by 6 cycles of postoperative chemotherapy, followed by XZ-C immunoregulatory Chinese medicine to enhance the long-term curative effect, and insist on long-term small-dose medication. It has been 6 years and is in good health.

Seven. Some typical cases of adjuvant treatment after rectal cancer

Case 44

Yan XXX, female,71 years old, teacher, in Wuhan
Medical record number: XXXX

Diagnosis:

Ascending colon cancer

The Figure of Diagnosis and treatment of ascending colon cancer is as the following :

1994. 12.19	1995. 7.4	1996	1997	1998	1999	2000	2001	2002	2003
Surgery	XZ-C	XZ-C	XZ-C	XZ-C	XZ-C	XZ-C	XZ-C	XZ-C	XZ-C

Serve XZ-C1+4

Medical history and treatment:

Due to abdominal pain and bloody stools, colon cancer was found under fiber colonoscopy (diagnosed by biopsy).

On December 19, 1994, he underwent radical resection of the right hemicolon. The pathology was that the colon was invaded by the serous membrane of the differentiated adenocarcinoma.

No other treatment was done after the operation. Came to the clinic on July 4, 1995. It was to adopt XZ-C1+4 immuno-regulatory anti-cancer traditional Chinese medicine as a postoperative adjuvant treatment to prevent postoperative metastasis and recurrence.

After taking XZ-C immune traditional Chinese medicine for a long time, it has been 10 years after the operation, and he is in good health. Followed up in April 2005, the old man was 81 years old, a healthy old man, and he played cards in the afternoon. See the above Figure.

Analysis and evaluation:

In this case, after resection of ascending colon cancer, he simply took XZ-C immuno-regulatory Chinese medicine for postoperative adjuvant treatment to strengthen the body to eliminate evil and prevent metastasis and recurrence. It has been 10 years after the operation and the condition is good.

This example prompts:

After surgery, supplemented with XZ-C immunomodulatory Chinese medicine treatment, **it can strengthen the body to eliminate evil, which can effectively prevent recurrence and metastasis.**

Case 45

Yin XXX, female, 60 years old, Huang Poren, Medical record number: XXXX

Diagnosis:

Sigmoid colon cancer, after left hemicolectomy

The Figure of Treatment after left colectomy for sigmoid colon cancer is as the following:

1999. 12.3	2000. 1.12	2001	2002	2003	2004	2005
Surgery	XZ-C	XZ-C	XZ-C	XZ-C	XZ-C	XZ-C

XZ-C1+4, LMS

Medical history and treatment:

In August 1998, the stool was bloody, and the local treatment was based on "hemorrhoids".

A colonoscopy was performed at Xiehe Hospital in October 1999, and there was a circular stenosis at 32 cm of the lens.

On December 3, 1999, the left colon was excised in Union Hospital. Pathology: papillary tubular adenocarcinoma of the sigmoid colon, invading the entire thickness of the intestinal wall, metastasis to mesenteric lymph nodes (6/8).

Came to Shuguang Clinic on January 12, 2000 to take XZ-C immune-regulated anti-cancer Chinese medicine, XZ-C1+4, LMS, MDZ, VT to prevent recurrence and metastasis, and take XZ-C immune-regulated anti-cancer Chinese medicine for 3 years. 8 months old.

On August 4, 2003, his son came to fetch medicine. He said that he was in good condition, doing housework every day, and was in a good mood. He brought more than 10 buckets of water every day to water the flowers and planted various flowers in a large yard.

I have grown some vegetables, and I have good spirits and appetite. The patient has always been in a good mood, optimistic mood, and good labor.

The patient always adhere to the XZ-C immune regulation Chinese medicine, take the medicine on time and in the amount every day. This patient did not receive adjuvant chemotherapy after surgery, and was simply taking XZ-C immune traditional Chinese medicine, which was an adjuvant therapy after surgery. The patient continued to take the XZ-C drug for another 4 months, and it had been 5 and a half years before the follow-up visit. See the above picture.

Analysis and evaluation:

This patient has sigmoid colon cancer and mesenteric lymph node metastasis. After radical surgery, WBC declines and cannot be assisted with chemotherapy. He is treated with XZ-C immunoregulatory anti-cancer traditional Chinese medicine so as to protect Thymus and to increase immune function, to protect bone marrow and to produce blood to improve the body's anti-cancer immunity so that it is to prevent metastasis and recurrence. It has been 5 and a half years since the follow-up visit, and the condition is generally good.

Case 46

Yu XXX, Female,63-year-old, cadre from Jilin
Medical record number: XXXX

Diagnosis:

Rectal adenocarcinoma

The Figure of Diagnosis and treatment of rectal adenocarcinoma is as the following:

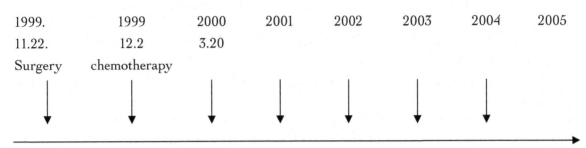

1999.　　　1999　　2000　　2001　　2002　　2003　　2004　　2005
11.22.　　　12.2　　3.20
Surgery　chemotherapy

WBC drops to 0.06 x 109/L

Medical history and treatment:

In October 1999, he had blood in the stool. The rectal microscope examined a large cauliflower-like mass on the finger 10 cm from the anus. The biopsy pathological section showed rectal adenocarcinoma.

On November 22, 1999, he underwent a radical resection of rectal cancer in the Affiliated Hospital with Dixon operation and recovered well.

The patient had Intraperitoneal chemotherapy on December 2 (fluorouricine 1.0g, 1/d, continuous use of 5d, carboplatin 100mg, 1/d, continuous use of 3d),

On December 9th, the white blood cell count dropped to 0.09X109/L,

On December 10, the white blood cell count dropped to 0.06X 109/L, and the white blood cell count rose to 1.1X109/L after 5 days of injection of the white blood cell-enhancing drug, lung infection, and persistent high fever of 40C.

On January 2, 2000, the patient took Tynene + ciprofloxacin, but the fever still persists, and the patient's throat is infected with 3 kinds of bacteria. The patient can't eat or drink water.

After taking "Dafukang" (Fuconwa) for 5 days, the body temperature dropped to 38C. The patient had pulmonary heart disease, high blood pressure and mild diabetes. At this point, the patient was extremely weakened and was in critical condition. He was critically ill twice. He got better after 2 months of treatment.

On March 20, 2000, the patient came to the anti-cancer clinic of Integrative Chinese and Western Medicine and treated with XZ-C immunomodulatory Chinese medicine. After 2 months of taking XZ-C1+4+LMS, the patient's appetite and general condition improved. The patient can get up. After half a year with take XZ-C medicine, the general condition has improved significantly, and he can take care of himself and do some housework. The recovery in September 2000 was very good. The patient can go to the nearby vegetable market to buy vegetables and do some light housework.

The patient has been taking XZ-C immune-regulating and control Chinese medicine daily for 5 years without interruption.

In May 2005, his daughter came to the outpatient clinic to collect the medicine, saying that the patient's health was recovering well. He was 68 years old at the time of follow-up. Do some housework, just like other healthy elderly people. See the above Figure.

Analysis and evaluation:

In this patient, after radical resection of rectal cancer and intraperitoneal chemotherapy, the body's immune function and bone marrow hematopoietic function were severely suppressed, which caused serious infection of the throat and both lungs, followed by a double fungal infection.

After treatment, the patient continued to take immuno-regulating –control Chinese medicine for a longer period of time.

XZ-C1 only inhibits cancer cells, does not affect normal cells, and strengthens the body.

XZ- C4 protects Thymus and increases immune function and promotes immunity, protects bone marrow, and promotes the recovery of overall immune function.

Chemotherapy cytotoxic drugs inhibit bone marrow, which actually leads to varying degrees of bone marrow aplasia. **The effect can sometimes last as long as 2-3 years.**

Therefore, the XZ-C immunomodulatory drug that protects the Thymus and protects the marrow and produces blood needs to be taken for several years. In order to facilitate the complete recovery of immune function and bone marrow hematopoietic function.

Case 47

Qian, male, 66 years old, from Wuhan, senior accountant
Medical record number: XXXX

Diagnosis:

Rectal adenocarcinoma

The Figure of Diagnosis and treatment of rectal adenocarcinoma is as the following:

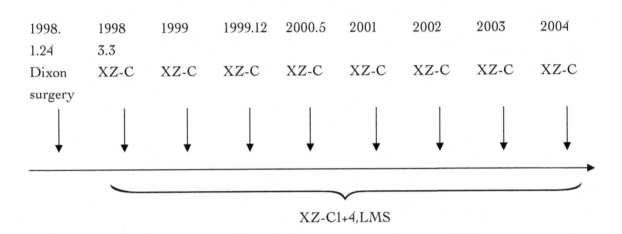

1998. 1.24	1998 3.3	1999	1999.12	2000.5	2001	2002	2003	2004
Dixon surgery	XZ-C	XZ-C	XZ-C	XZ-C	XZ-C	XZ-C	XZ-C	XZ-C

XZ-C1+4,LMS

Medical history and treatment conditions:

intermittent diarrhea, constipation for 2 years, stool with blood, anal digital examination of the knee and chest at 6 points to touch a 3cmX 3cm mass.

On January 20, 1998, fiber colonoscopy showed malignant transformation of rectal polyps.

A Dixon operation was performed in Union Hospital on January 24, 1998. The colon was removed 40 cm. The pathological section was a rectal tubular adenocarcinoma, which was moderately differentiated and invaded the superficial muscle layer of the intestinal wall.

No lymph node metastasis was seen, and no cancer cells were seen at the cut end. No chemotherapy was done after surgery,

Came to the outpatient clinic on March 3, 1998, treated with XZ-C immunomodulatory Chinese medicine alone, and took XZ-C medicine for a long time for nearly 8 years.

He has been back to work for 5 years without discomfort. Continue to take XZ-C immune regulation Chinese medicine. See the above Figure.

Analysis and evaluation:

This patient was a rectal adenocarcinoma. The pathological section of the patient underwent Dixon radical resection in January 1998 to be a rectal tubular adenocarcinoma, moderately differentiated, **no chemotherapy after surgery, and XZ-Cl+4 immunoregulatory Chinese medicine alone as a postoperative adjuvant The treatment has been in good condition for the past 8 years.**

This example prompts:

After radical resection of rectal cancer, Dixon surgery, chemotherapy was not used, and XZ-C immunoregulatory Chinese medicine was used only. It protects Thymus and promotes immunity, protects the marrow to produces blood, improves the postoperative immune level, strengthens the patient's disease resistance, improves the quality of life, and prevents recurrence and metastasis. The patient is in good condition.

Case 48

Yang**, female, 32 years old, from Zaoyang, accountant
Medical record number: XXXX

Diagnosis:

Rectal villous tubular adenocarcinoma

The Figure of Diagnosis and treatment process of rectal villous tubular adenocarcinoma is as the following:

1997. 9. 17	1997. 12	1999	2000	2001	2002	2003	2004
Surgery	XZ-C	XZ-C	XZ-C	XZ-C	XZ-C	XZ-C	XZ-C

XZ-Cl+4

Medical history and treatment:

The stool was bloody, and the biopsy of the rectal microscope in September 1997 was rectal cancer.

Radical resection of rectal cancer was performed on September 17, 1997.

The tumor was 4cm from the anus and the base was about 1.0cmX 1.0cm in size. The postoperative pathological report was rectal villous tubular adenocarcinoma, which invaded the tube wall and the entire thickness, and metastasized to mesenteric lymph nodes.. Chemotherapy was performed once after surgery, but no more chemotherapy was done because of the significant decrease in white blood cells.

On December 3, 1997, he came to the outpatient clinic of the Anti-cancer Cooperation Group of Integrated Traditional Chinese and Western Medicine and used XZ-C immune control Chinese medicine treatment.

After taking XZ-C1+4, the general condition is good and the blood condition has recovered. After taking XZ-C traditional Chinese medicine for 8 years, he has not undergone other radiotherapy or chemotherapy, and he is in a good state of anxiety and recovery, and doing housework as normal. See the above Figure.

Analysis and evaluation:

This patient underwent a radical resection of rectal cancer on September 17, 1997. During the operation, mesenteric lymph node metastasis was seen.

The cancer invaded the entire thickness of the bowel wall. Chemotherapy was performed once after the operation, and the response was big, so the patient didn't do it again.

From December 3, 1997, the patient came to the Shuguang Oncology Clinic of the Chinese and Western Medicine and Anti-Cancer Cooperation Group, and used XZ-C immune regulation anti-cancer Chinese medicine as a postoperative adjuvant treatment to prevent postoperative recurrence and metastasis. The patient takes long-term medication for 8 years. The healthy recovery is good.

Case 49

Chen XXX, female, 68 years old, chief physician.
Medical record number: XXXX

Diagnosis:

Colon cancer

The Figure of Diagnosis and treatment of colon cancer is as the following:

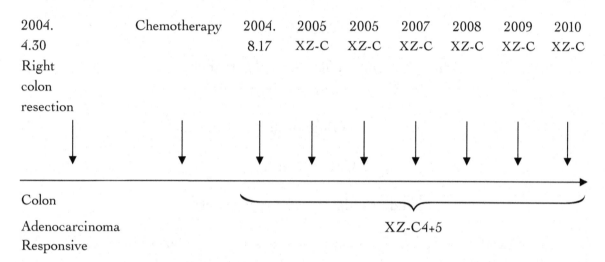

Medical history and treatment:

The acute intestinal obstruction could not be relieved after treatment. On April 30, 2004, he was investigated in the emergency operation of Xinhua Hospital. It was found that a cecum mass was found and the right hemicolectomy was performed. Postoperative pathology: Colonic papillary adenocarcinoma with obstruction.

There was once postoperative chemotherapy and the patient had large response, intolerable, came to Shuguang Oncology Clinic on August 17, 2004, using XZ-C immunoregulatory Chinese medicine as postoperative adjuvant treatment.

After taking XZ-C4+5, the patient has a good appetite after taking the medicine. The patient comes to the clinic every month for follow-up visits, take medicine, and insist on taking it for a long time. It has been more than 6 years and my health is in good condition. See the above Figure.

Analysis and evaluation:

This patient had acute intestinal obstruction due to cecal tumor, emergency surgical exploration, right hemicolectomy, and a postoperative chemotherapy. The response was severe and could no longer be used. He came to the outpatient clinic to take XZ-C immunoregulatory anti-cancer medicine as an adjuvant treatment after surgery.

He insisted on taking small amounts of medicine for a long time and visiting the outpatient clinic every month to get medicine. It has been more than 6 years so far, and he is generally in good condition. He is a healthy old man.

Case 50

Zhang**, female, 38 years old, Hanchuan.
Medical record number: XXXX

Diagnosis:

Colon cancer

Medical history and treatment:

Intermittent abdominal pain for 5 months, colonoscopy revealed a raised lesion of the descending colon. Left hemicolectomy + right ovarian resection was performed on October 4, 2005. Postoperative pathology: a poorly differentiated adenocarcinoma and mesenteric in the descending colon, Right ovarian metastasis.

The patient had 6 cycles of postoperative chemotherapy, then came to the Shuguang Oncology Clinic on August 18, 2006, taking XZ-C immune-regulating and control anti-cancer Chinese medicine, continuous consolidation therapy, taking XZ-C1.4+LMS+MDZ, long-term adherence to medication, and monthly follow-up visits to the outpatient clinic for medicine. It has been 5 years so far, and his health has recovered well.

Case 51

Long xxxx, male, 60 years old, from Sichuan, professor
Medical record number: XXXX

Diagnosis:

Rectal cancer

The figure of diagnosis and treatment of rectal cancer is as the following:

2000. 3.2	2000. 03	2000. 4 5.30	2000.	2001	2002	2003	2004	2005	2006	2007	2008	2009
Rectal Cancer Radical resection	radiotherapy x12	Chemo once	XZ-C	XZ-C	XZ-C	XZ-C	XZ-C	XZ-C	XZ-C	XZ-C	XZ-C	XZ-C

XZ-C1+4+LMS+MDZ

Medical history and treatment:

In November 1999, he had blood in the stool and was treated as "hemorrhoids".

In February 2000, he was diagnosed as rectal cancer by a rectal biopsy.

Radical resection of rectal cancer was performed in Tongji Hospital on March 2, 2000. The patient had Mile's procedure, postoperative pathology: rectal moderately differentiated adenocarcinoma.

Patient had postoperative radiotherapy 12 times, chemotherapy once,

then came to Shuguang Cancer Specialist Clinic to take XZ-C1+4+LMS+M DZ on May 30, 2000.

After taking the medicine, the patient has a good appetite. The patient insists on taking a small amount of medicine for a long period of time. It has been 10 years since the follow-up visits and medicines were taken. He is in good health and all the top indicators are normal. See the above Figure.

Analysis and evaluation:

This patient had a radical cure for rectal cancer with Mile's operation, 13 radiotherapy and 1 chemotherapy after the operation. After that, Immune-regulating and control Chinese medicine was used as an adjuvant treatment after the operation, which Thymus was promoted and the bone marrow was protected for blood production. He insisted on long-term medication and came to the clinic every month. After taking the medicine, the general condition is good, and the appetite is good. It has been 10 years and the health condition is good.

6. Some typical cases of postoperative adjuvant treatment of gallbladder cancer

Case 52

Song xxx, male, 51 years old, from Tianmen, cadre
Medical record number: XXXX

Diagnosis:

Tubular adenocarcinoma of the lower common bile duct

The Figure of Diagnosis and treatment of tubular adenocarcinoma in the lower part of the common bile duct is as the following:

2003.9	Chemotherapy x3 times	2003.11	2004	2005	2006	2007	2008	2009	2010
Pancreaticoduodenum		XZ-C	XZ-C	XZ-C	XZ-C	XZ-C	XZ-C	XZ-C	XZ-C

→

Lower end of common bile duct XZ-C1+4+5+LMS+MDZ
Tubular adenocarcinoma Ampulla tumor

Medical history and treatment:

Painless jaundice for a week, local CT examination showed tumor of ampulla.

On September 7, 2003, Professor Qian was asked to perform pancreaticoduodenectomy at Jianghan Oilfield Central Hospital in Qianjiang City. The operation went smoothly and the size of the tumor was as the size of finger. Pathology: (Lower section of common bile duct) Tubular adenocarcinoma (high grade one with medium differentiation) invaded the entire thickness of the tube wall and the head of the pancreas.

After the second postoperative chemotherapy, the patient came to the Shuguang Oncology Specialist Clinic to take XZ-C immune regulation and control anti-cancer Chinese medicine, XZ-C1+4+5+LMS+MDZ+Vit, continue to complete the chemotherapy process, that is, chemotherapy + immunomodulatory drugs, complete chemotherapy 6 Continue to take XZ-C4+5 to protect Thymus and increase immune function, and to protect bone marrow and to product blood for a long period of time. After taking the medicine, the mental appetite is good, and the general condition is good. So far, he has been taking XZ-C immunoregulatory Chinese medicine for 7 years. The general condition is good, the health condition is good, and he has been back to work for three years. He is strong and healthy. See the above Figure.

Analysis and evaluation:

This patient underwent pancreaticoduodenectomy for ampullary tumors. After several chemotherapy treatments, he insisted on taking XZ-C immunoregulatory Chinese medicine for a long time to protect the Thymus and to increase immune function, to protect bone marrow and to promote blood production to control recurrence. Transfer, take XZ-C1+4+5 daily for the first three years, and then take XZ-C4+5 for a long time. Now for 7 years, she is still taking the medicine and is in good health.

Why are you still taking medicine for so many years?

Because the biological characteristics of cancer cells are constantly dividing, proliferating, and likely to recur and metastasize, postoperative adjuvant therapy should also be accompanied by long-term treatment, to have Thymus protection and increase immunity, protection of thymus function, and long-term increase immunity.

This example prompts:

XZ-C immunoregulatory Chinese medicine can be used for postoperative adjuvant treatment after pancreaticoduodenectomy. This patient has been taking long-term medication after surgery for more than 7 years, and his health has recovered well.

Case 53

Dai XXX, female, 59 years old, Wuhan
Medical Record Number: xxxx

Diagnosis:

Gallbladder adenocarcinoma

The Figure of Treatment of gallbladder cancer cases is as the following:

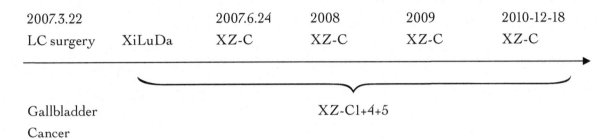

2007.3.22		2007.6.24	2008	2009	2010-12-18
LC surgery	XiLuDa	XZ-C	XZ-C	XZ-C	XZ-C

Gallbladder
Cancer

XZ-C1+4+5

Medical history and treatment:

Due to the physical examination of gallbladder stones, LC cholecystectomy was performed at Zhongshan Hospital of Zhejiang Province on March 22, 2007. After the operation, the thickness of the bottom wall of the gallbladder of the specimen was about 1.8cm, and the range was 2.5 X 3cm. Pathological section: well-differentiated adenocarcinoma, immunohistochemical CK (++), CEA (+).

On March 30, 2007, gastroscopy showed chronic erosive gastritis, bile reflux gastritis, Hp (+), and oral Xeloda after operation.

On June 24, 2007, the patient came to Shuguang Oncology Clinic to take XZ-C immune-regulating and control anti-cancer traditional Chinese medicine as an adjuvant treatment after operation, orally take XZ-C1 +XZ-C4 +XZ-C5 +LMS+MDZ and treat Helicobacter pylori.

After take medicine for one month, the spirit and appetite recovered well, and he insisted on XZ-C immune regulation and control Chinese medicine for Thymus protection and increasing immunity. So far, he has been in good health for nearly 4 years. See the above Figure.

Evaluation:

This patient is gallbladder cancer, diagnosed as gallbladder stones before surgery, cholecystectomy under laparoscopic surgery, postoperative gallbladder pathology is well-differentiated adenocarcinoma, postoperative Xeloda two courses of treatment, XZ-C immune regulation and control anti-cancer medicine for postoperative adjuvant treatment, the patient has been taking it for a long time for nearly 4 years. The patient has good appetite and good health.

Case 54

Gong**, male, 57 years old, Wuhan Medical Record Number: xxxx

Diagnosis:

Gallbladder moderately differentiated adenocarcinoma

The Figure of Treatment of gallbladder cancer cases is as the following:

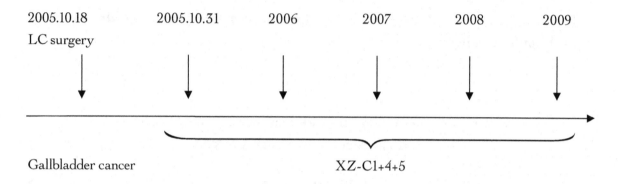

Medical history and treatment:

In September 2005, the upper abdomen had a dull pain, and the examination was a gallbladder polyp.

Laparoscopic cholecystectomy was performed at a Wuhan hospital on October 18, 2009. The pathological report after the operation was moderately differentiated gallbladder cancer.

On October 28, 2005, the MR report showed no obvious metastases in the liver and no postoperative radiotherapy and chemotherapy were performed.

The patient came to the Shuguang Oncology Clinic on October 31, 2005, and took XZ-C1+4+5+LMS+MDZ and other immunomodulation as adjuvant postoperative treatment. After taking the medicine, the general condition recovered well and the spirit and appetite were good. The patient insisted on taking XZ-C Immune regulation and control Chinese medicine for a long time and has been in good health for more than 5 years. See the above Figure.

Evaluation:

This patient has gallbladder cancer, which was diagnosed as gallbladder entrapped and the gallbladder was removed under laparoscopic surgery. The postoperative pathology was gallbladder cancer. Due to the early discovery, no radiotherapy or chemotherapy was performed after the operation, and the XZ-X immunomodulatory anti-cancer Chinese medicine was used as an adjuvant treatment after the operation. The long-term medication has been used for 3 years, and the health is restored as normal.

7. **Some typical cases of postoperative adjuvant treatment such as kidney cancer and bladder cancer**

Case 55

Chen xxx, male, 62 years old, senior engineer, Wuhan, Medical record number: XXXX

Diagnosis:

Right kidney Meng tumor, bladder cancer recurrence after surgery

The Figure of Treatment of right renal pelvis tumor, bladder cancer recurrence after surgery was as the following:

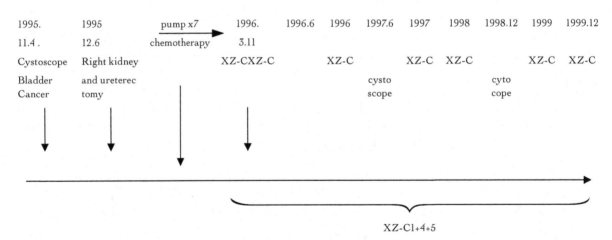

Medical **history and treatment**:

Hematuria for 2 years, cystoscopy on November 4, 1995, confirmed as bladder cancer,

On November 21, 1995 CT found a tumor of the right renal pelvis,

On December 6, 1995, he underwent right kidney and ureter resection, bladder sleeve resection, and 7 postoperative local infusion chemotherapy.

On March 8, 1996, the cystoscope was re-examined, and it was found that there was a rigid bulge on the left side of the bladder to prevent recurrence.

On March 11, 1996, he came to the outpatient clinic of the cooperative group to use XZ-Cl +4+6 immunoregulatory Chinese medicine alone. After taking the medicine, both the spirit and appetite improved.

The cystoscope was reviewed on June 24, 1996. The surface was smooth and the new organisms had disappeared. He continued to take XZ-C Chinese medicine for a long time for immune control to prevent recurrence and metastasis. Until June 11, 1997, there was no abnormality in the cystoscope.

On December 28, 1998, there was no abnormality in the cystoscopy.

The follow-up visit on June 26, 1999 was in good condition. The patient had been taking XZ-Cl+4+6 daily for 10 years, which prevented the recurrence or metastasis of bladder tumors.

The patient returned on May 6, 2005, and the patient was in good condition. He has completely returned to a normal healthy elderly. See the above Figure.

Analysis and evaluation:

This patient had a recurrence of bladder cancer after surgery. He has insisted on taking xz-c immune regulation Chinese medicine for more than 10 years.

The recurrence or metastasis of bladder cancer has been stopped, and the condition is good. After repeated inspections of the cystoscopy, it has completely returned to normal.

This example prompts:

XZ-C immunomodulatory Chinese medicine can improve the patient's immune function, promote the stability, control and disappearance of primary and recurrence cancer, and prevent the recurrence and metastasis of bladder cancer. The patient's health is in good condition,

Case 56

Ling** Male 68-year-old professor from Wuhan
Medical record number: XXXX

Diagnosis:

Recurrence of bladder cancer after surgery

The Figure of the treatment process of bladder cancer recurrence after surgery is as the following:

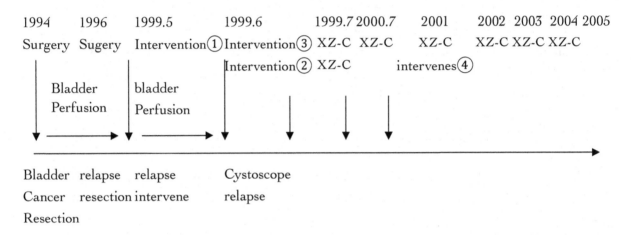

Medical history and treatment:

In April 1994, he underwent bladder cancer resection at the Provincial People's Hospital. The disease was checked for transitional cell carcinoma. After bladder perfusion chemotherapy, MMC was stopped due to a significant decrease in white blood cells.

At the beginning of 1996, it was checked for recurrence, and 8 tumors in the bladder were removed again. After the operation, the bladder is infused twice a month. After 3 months with phagetepa+5-FU, stop for 3 months and then do it for 3 months.

It is twice a month, until the beginning of 1997.

In May 1998, there was flocculation in the cystoscopy at Union Hospital. In December, the B-ultrasound re-examination was cystitis.

In April 1999, he underwent cystoscopy due to hematuria. A 4cm² tumor was found in the triangle area. CT and biopsy showed that the results were all bladder cancer.

In May 1999, he underwent interventional bladder arterial chemotherapy perfusion.

In June, the patient did the second infusion of fluorourea + mitomycin + carboplatin (5-FU+MMC+carboplatin). After blood transfusion, the white blood cells decreased to 2X109/L.

In September, the patient did the third infusion of fluorourea+ mitomycin + camptothecin, the white blood cell count dropped to 1.2X109/L, it was injected with Gilifen Shengbai needle.

Past history:

In 1992, the stroke was over, high blood pressure (160/90mmHg), diabetes.

He suffered from hepatitis in 1984 and cirrhosis in 1998.

Family history:

The second brother (after hepatitis B) has liver cancer, and the younger brother has rectal cancer

When the patient came to the clinic in July 1999, the blood picture was low after being treated, so the patient used Husui Shengxue Decoction and X-C1 + XZ-C4 + XZ-C6 Chinese medicine to promote anti-cancer. The whole blood picture rose to normal after taking the medicine for 6 months. The spirit and appetite also improved significantly, continue to take the medicine.

In July 2000, cystoscopy showed that the bladder was well filled, and a 1.3cmX0.6cm medium echo light cluster was seen in the triangle area. It was considered as a recurrent tumor. He continued to take the medicine until June 2001. He had frequent urination due to prostate hyperplasia. CT review of bladder lesions was larger than before (compared with February 1999), and bladder artery intervention was performed once.

Continue to take XZ-C1 +XZ-C4 +XZ-C until July 6, 2002 to review the bladder CT, the bladder cancer lesion is smaller than before, after taking the drug, the general condition is good, the appetite is good, and there is no hematuria. It has been 6 years at the time of follow-up, The control of the lesion is stable, no further development, and no distant metastasis. See the above Figure.

Analysis and evaluation:

This patient is a transitional cell carcinoma of the bladder. After resection, it has recurred many times. Long-term infusion chemotherapy failed to prevent the recurrence. Due to bladder perfusion and multiple cystoscopy for many years, as well as prostatic hyperplasia and urethra stricture, cystoscopy is difficult to perform.

Long-term use of XZ-C immunomodulatory anti-cancer medicine XZ-C1+4+6, bladder neoplasms have not developed, no metastasis, 11 years since the onset of the disease to the follow-up visit, the general condition is good, the spirit and appetite are good, and the walking activities are long. Hematuria sometimes occurs.

Case 57

He * Male 76-year-old Henan cadre
Medical record number: XXXX

Diagnosis:

Clear cell carcinoma of the lower pole of the left kidney

The Figure of the treatment process of left renal clear cell carcinoma Is as the following:

2000.8.31	2000.9.28	2001	2002	2003	2004	2005
Surgery	XZ-C	XZ-C	XZ-C	XZ-C	XZ-C	XZ-C

XZ-C1+4+6

Medical history and treatment:

There were 200 renal cysts in 1996. The annual physical examination of the left kidney cyst was 7. 5cm X 6. 5cm, and CT and MRI examination showed that the left kidney was tumor.

The left nephrectomy was performed at Tongji Hospital on August 31, 2000.

The pathology report was moderately differentiated renal clear cell carcinoma. After surgery, he took medroxyprogesterone acetate without radiotherapy or chemotherapy.

He came to Shuguang Oncology Clinic on September 28, 2000, and used XZ-C1+4 +6 immune-regulated anti-cancer Chinese medicine to protect breasts and promote blood circulation and marrow. After taking the medicine for 1 month, the spirit is good, the sleep is good, and the appetite is lacking. After taking the medicine for 3 months, the general condition is good, the mental appetite is good, and the sleep is good. After 1 year of taking the medicine, he was rechecked. Abdominal B-ultrasound, chest X-ray film and various routine tests were all normal. Continue to take XZ-C1 + XZ-C4 + XZ-C6 immune-regulating Chinese medicine to prevent recurrence and metastasis. It has been 3 years since the follow-up visit, and the health condition has recovered well. The follow-up visit on April 10, 2005 is generally in good condition, with a red face, a loud voice, good energy, a little fat, and presbycusis. The health condition should be 100 according to the Kalok score. In addition, re-examination of CT, chest X-ray film, liver and gallbladder ultrasound, liver and kidney function, and blood biochemistry were all normal, except for an enlarged prostate. See the above Figure.

Analysis and evaluation:

This case is a clear cell carcinoma of the left kidney. He was 76 years old at the time of the operation. Due to his advanced age and frailty, he did not undergo postoperative radiotherapy and only used XZ-C immunoregulatory Chinese medicine. It was postoperative adjuvant treatment, breast protection and blood production. Improve overall immunity to prevent recurrence and metastasis. He has been taking XZ-C immunomodulatory drugs for a long time for 5 years. He was 80 years old at the time of follow-up. In general, he has good appetite, red face, energetic, loud voice, and is a healthy old man.

Case 58

Yu xxx, male, 69 years old, from Heilongjiang, cadre
Medical record number: XXXX

Diagnosis:

Transitional cell carcinoma of the bladder

The Figure of the treatment process of transitional cell carcinoma of the bladder is as the following:

1998.3	1998.5	1998	1999	2000	2001	2002	2003	2004
Operation	chemotherapyx1	XZ-C	XZ-C	XZ-C	XZ-C	XZ-C	XZ-C	CXZ-C

Medical history and treatment:

Hematuria was found on February 27, 1998, and on March 2, cystoscopy and B-ultrasound, a round mass was seen on the anterior wall of the bladder, with a size of 1.6cmX 1.4cm, protruding into the bladder cavity, which is a new organism on the anterior wall of the bladder.

After surgery on March 10, 1998, the tumor tissue in the bladder was removed. The pathological section showed transitional cell carcinoma of the bladder skin. The doctor informed that the tumor is prone to recurrence.

Postoperative chemotherapy was performed once (May 26, 1998). The reaction was severe, nausea, vomiting, and general malaise. The lift testicle was significantly enlarged, so the chemotherapy was stopped.

On June 18, 1998, the patient came to the Shuguang Oncology Clinic of the Anti-Cancer Cooperation Group of Integrated Traditional Chinese and Western Medicine, treated with XZ-C1+ +4+6, and came to the clinic for review every month. The general condition is good, the urine is normal, and no other treatment is used. It has been more than 6 years and no abnormalities have been seen. See the above Figure.

Analysis and evaluation:

In this case, surgery was performed on March 10, 1998, and 3 tumor tissues in the bladder were removed. The pathological section showed transitional cell carcinoma of the bladder. The postoperative chemotherapy was performed once, and the reaction was serious, but no chemotherapy was performed. June 18, 1998 the patient came to the outpatient clinic of the Anti-Cancer Collaborative Group of Integrated Traditional Chinese and Western Medicine, and was treated with XZ-C1+4+6 immune Chinese medicine. It has been more than 7 years at the time of follow-up. He is in good health and has not been treated by other methods, and no recurrence or metastasis has been seen.

Case 59

Zhong** Male 66-year-old Wuxi cadre
Medical record number: XXXX

Diagnosis:

Right kidney clear cell carcinoma, whole body bone metastasis, supraclavicular metastasis

The Figure of treatment of bone metastases from renal cancer is as the following:

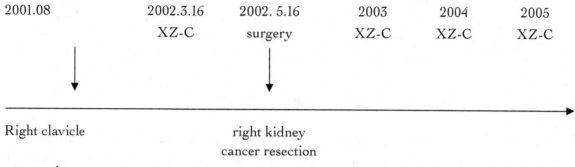

| 2001.08 | 2002.3.16 | 2002. 5.16 | 2003 | 2004 | 2005 |
| | XZ-C | surgery | XZ-C | XZ-C | XZ-C |

Right clavicle

right kidney

cancer resection

metastasis

L2, L4 bone metastasis

Medical history and treatment:

In August 2001, due to pain in the right shoulder, it was found to be "frozen shoulder" after examination.

Later, a large walnut mass appeared on the right clavicle near the sternum, and the puncture showed adenocarcinoma cells.

Through abdominal, chest B-ultrasound and CT, no primary tumor was found.

The patient came to Shuguang Oncology Clinic on March 16, 2002 for XZ-C immunomodulation and integrated traditional Chinese and Western medicine treatment.

The patient took XZ-CH4 internally and XZ-C3 externally. After the application, the clavicle mass became softer and slightly shrunk.

On March 24, 2002, B-ultrasound found a mass mass of 3.1cmX4.3cin in the right kidney area, CT: L2, L4 had bone destruction, XZ-Cl + XZ-C4 + XZ-C6 was used, and Gemcit -abine, GEM) + cisplatin chemotherapy for 1 course.

The right kidney resection was performed on May 16, 2002. The tumor of the right kidney was about the size of a table tennis ball. The pathological report was clear cell carcinoma. Due to immune regulation anticancer drugs, the general condition was good after taking the drug, and the appetite was good. Walking activities as usual, 2002.. 2003.. July 2004, come to the outpatient clinic for follow-up visits and medicines every month, and the mental appetite and condition are basically stable.

Until July 2004, suddenly dizzy, easy to forget to speak, and contradictory, CT examination was cerebral hemorrhage, staying in neurology, lying in bed for 3 weeks, CT re-detected blood has been absorbed, continue to take XZ-Cl +6 +2, LMS, Brucea javanica, agrimony granules, longkui granules, Huangmie granules, Huangqin granules, etc., the general condition gradually improved, and the spirit and appetite were better. See the above Figure.

Analysis and evaluation:

In August 2001, due to the discovery of a metastatic mass on the right clavicle and L2, L4 bone metastasis, this patient was punctured by the supraclavicular mass and was found to be a metastatic adenocarcinoma. After a comprehensive examination, he was found to be a tumor of the right kidney. He had a right kidney resection on May 16, 2002. For clear cell carcinoma, XZ-C immunomodulatory anti-cancer Chinese medicine was taken on March 16, 2002. After oral administration and external application, the condition was stable for more than 3 years, and no further metastasis was controlled. After taking the medicine, the patient had good appetite and stable condition.

Case 60

Xu** Male 61 years old Wuhan fitter
Medical record number: XXXX

Diagnosis:

Left kidney clear cell carcinoma

The Figure of Diagnosis and treatment of left renal clear cell carcinoma is as the following:

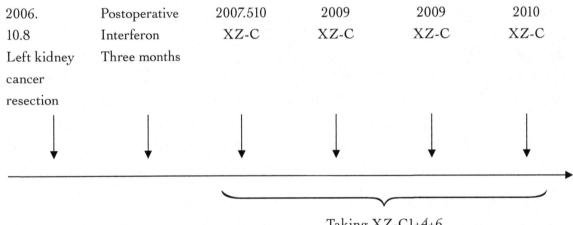

| 2006.
10.8
Left kidney
cancer
resection | Postoperative
Interferon
Three months | 2007.510
XZ-C | 2009
XZ-C | 2009
XZ-C | 2010
XZ-C |

Taking XZ-Cl+4+6

Medical history and treatment:

Physical examination on October 27, 2006, B-ultrasound found a mass in the left kidney

On November 8, 2006, Professor Tongji was invited to perform a left nephrectomy at the Wuhan Iron and Steel General Hospital. Postoperative pathology: clear cell carcinoma, lymph nodes (0/2), postoperative interferon and IL-2 treatment for 3 months, there is no Chemotherapy.

On May 10, 2007, the patient came to Shuguang Oncology Specialty Clinic to take xz-c immunomodulation adjuvant therapy, use XZ-C1+4+6, LMS and MDZ for continuous long-term medication, and come to the specialist clinic for follow-up visits and medicines every month. It has been 4 years, generally in good condition, healthy and strong, and is a healthy old man. See the above Figure.

Analysis and evaluation:

This patient was left renal clear cell carcinoma. He did not undergo radiotherapy or chemotherapy after surgery. He took XZ-C immunomodulatory Chinese medicine as adjuvant treatment after surgery. He has been taking XZ-C immunomodulatory Chinese medicine for more than 4 years. He is in good condition and has been reviewed repeatedly. The patient has completely recovered as a healthy old man.

This example prompts:

XZ-C immune regulation Chinese medicine can improve the patient's immune function and prevent recurrence and metastasis.

Case 61

Shi * * Female 61 years old from Hunan
Medical record number: XXXX

Diagnosis:

Renal cell carcinoma

The Figure of Diagnosis and treatment of renal cell carcinoma is as the following:

2006.10		2007.9	2008	2009	2010.11.14
Partial left kidney resection	Chemotherapyx2	XZ-C	XZ-C	XZ-C	XZ-C

Renal cell carcinoma

XZ-C1+4+6+LMS+V it

Medical history and treatment:

Physical examination in early October 2006 revealed a mass in the right kidney, which was asymptomatic.

The right kidney mass was removed (partial nephrectomy) in October 2006, and the postoperative pathology was renal cell carcinoma.

He had undergone chemotherapy after surgery. In September 2007, he came to Shuguang Oncology Clinic to take XZ-C immune-regulating and control anti-cancer Chinese medicine for postoperative adjuvant treatment. He took XZ-C1+4+6+LMS+Vit for a long time. It has been 4 years for follow-up visits and medicine collection every month and is in good health. See the above Figure.

Analysis and evaluation:

This patient's right kidney mass was partially nephrectomy, and the postoperative pathology was renal cell carcinoma. In September 2007, he came to the specialist clinic to take XZ1+4+6+LMS as an adjuvant treatment after the operation. He has been taking medication for a long time and has been taking medicine for more than 4 years. The patient is in good health.

8. **Some typical cases of postoperative adjuvant treatment such as thyroid cancer and retroperitoneal tumors**

Case 62

Peng XXX, female, 39 years old from Leshan, Sichuan Cadre
Medical record number: XXXX

Diagnosis:

Thyroid cancer

The figure of diagnosis and treatment of Thyroid cancer is as the following:

1999.05	1999.07	2000	2001	2002	2003	2004	2005.05
Thyroid Surgery	XZ-C	XZ-C	XZ-C	XZ-C	XZ-C	XZ-C	followup

Medical history and treatment:

The right neck mass was removed on April 27, 1999, and the postoperative examination was (thyroid) follicular papillary carcinoma with focal lymphocytic thyroiditis.

Radical thyroid cancer surgery was performed on May 6, 1999.

After the operation, the voice was hoarse, but radiotherapy and chemotherapy were not performed.

Came to Shuguang Oncology Clinic on July 24, 1999 to take XZ-C immunomodulatory Chinese medicine XZ-C1+XZ-C4, LMS, VS postoperative adjuvant treatment, monthly follow-up visits, continuous XZ-C immunomodulatory medicine for half a year,

By January 2000, the voice gradually improved, and after another 3 months of taking XZ-C, the voice gradually returned to normal.

The general condition is good, the mental appetite is good, the physical strength is restored, and he resumes work. He insists on taking XZ1+4 for a long time to improve the overall immune function. It has been 6 years since the follow-up visit, and the follow-up visit in May 2005 is in good health. See the above Figure.

Analysis and evaluation:

This case is thyroid follicular papillary carcinoma. Severe hoarseness occurred after radical resection. No postoperative adjuvant treatments such as radiotherapy and chemotherapy were performed. XZ-C immunoregulatory Chinese medicine was simply taken orally as adjuvant treatment after surgery to improve overall immune function, prevent recurrence and metastasis.

Case 63

Cheng** Male 64-year-old cadre from Xinzhou,
Hubei Medical record number: xxxx

Diagnosis:

Retroperitoneal tumor

The figure of the treatment process of retroperitoneal tumors is as the following:

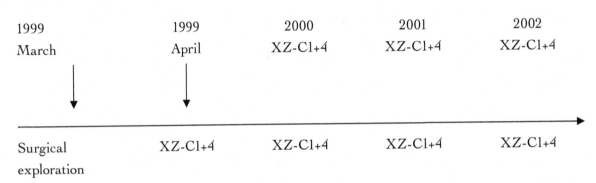

1999	1999	2000	2001	2002
March	April	XZ-C1+4	XZ-C1+4	XZ-C1+4
Surgical exploration	XZ-C1+4	XZ-C1+4	XZ-C1+4	XZ-C1+4

Medical history and treatment:

On January 6, 1999, there was sudden chest discomfort, pain, and vomiting. The emergency department considered it to be "acute gastroenteritis", the surgical consultation suspected pancreatitis, and the gastroscopy on March 3 showed duodenal obstruction.

Laparotomy on March 6, 1999 showed that the retroperitoneal tumor was wrapped in large blood vessels. During the operation, a 6cm X 9cm mass was found at the root of the small mesentery. It was hard, fixed, and had an uneven surface. It was tightly adhered to the abdominal aorta and superior mesenteric artery and compressed. The transverse part of the duodenum is difficult to remove, but the proximal end of the duodenum is anastomosed with Rou x-y of the jejunum. The tumor cannot be removed. Therefore, a combination of Chinese and Western medicine is ordered.

On April 4, 1999, Shuguang Oncology Specialist Clinic started to take XZ-C1+4 immunoregulatory anti-cancer Chinese medicine. The patient started to take XZ-C1+4 Chinese medicine continuously on May 1999 until February 2002. During this period, the patient performed irregular outpatient rechecks and medicines, and my health was good. See the above Figure.

Analysis and evaluation:

This patient was found to be a retroperitoneal tumor by laparotomy on March 6, 1999. The large blood vessels were tightly wrapped around the roots of the mesentery and could not be resected, and he did not dare to take slices. However, judging from the hardness, fixed, and uneven surface, it should be a malignant tumor. After taking XZ-C traditional Chinese medicine for 4 years in the cancer specialist clinic, the condition is stable, has not developed or metastasized, and the current health status is still good.

Case 64

Qi** Female 67-year-old worker from Shijiazhuang City
Medical record number: XXXX

Diagnosis:

Postoperative recurrence of peritoneal tumor

The Figure of the treatment process of postoperative recurrence of abdominal cat liquid tumor is as the following:

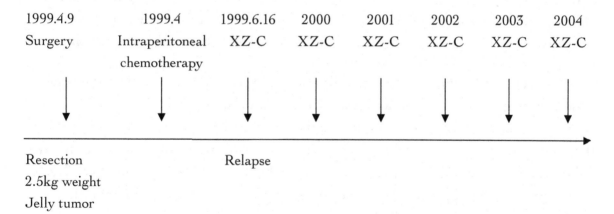

1999.4.9	1999.4	1999.6.16	2000	2001	2002	2003	2004
Surgery	Intraperitoneal chemotherapy	XZ-C	XZ-C	XZ-C	XZ-C	XZ-C	XZ-C

Resection
2.5kg weight
Jelly tumor

Relapse

Medical history and treatment:

Due to growing abdomen and ascites, the patient was admitted to Tongji Hospital in March 1999. Ascites sign++, frog belly, palpable intra-abdominal mass.

On April 9 laparotomy: the abdominal cavity was filled with jelly-like masses of varying sizes, one by one they were excised, weighing 2.5 kg, **5-FU 500 mg was**

placed during the operation, and chemotherapy was placed in the abdominal cavity.

From the 4th day after the operation, 5-FU 500mg was injected once a day for 5 days and carboplatin 100mg once a day for 3 days.

Came to the Shuguang Oncology Clinic on June 16, 1999, and took the XZ-C immunomodulatory anti-cancer Chinese medicine XZ-C1+4. After taking the medicine for 2 months, the spirit and appetite were good, and the weight gained. Physical examination: unbuckled and abnormal supraclavicular, flat and soft abdomen, unbuckled and abnormal, ascites (1), continue to take XZ-C immunoregulatory Chinese medicine for a long time, and come to the outpatient clinic every month to get the medicine until November 26, 2000 At the follow-up visit, the upper middle abdomen can be buckled and the fist mass of about adults can be buckled during the physical examination. It is hard, with multiple nodules on the surface, deep fixation, and clear borders. It is a recurrence of abdominal tumor after surgery. The patient's family refused to have the operation for the patient and also refuse chemotherapy so that the patient continues to take XZ-C immune regulation Chinese medicine XZ-C+4, LMS, MDZ, and apply XZ-C3 anti-cancer swelling ointment externally. The patient continues to take the medicine every day until February 24, 2002. Physical examination at the return visit: the supraclavicular is not buckled and abnormal, the abdomen Soft, large lumps that can be buckled into the fist, hard in quality, deep fixed, with clear edges, **but smaller than before, and the condition is stable.**

As of December 15, 2004, the re-examination for physical examination, the general condition is good, the mental appetite is good, but the abdomen is bulging, ascites sign++, the abdomen can be buttoned and the adult fist is large, the surface is uneven, the feeling of nodules, deep fixation, there was no signs of metastasis. After the addition of Xiaoshui Decoction, the ascites subsided, and the patient took XZ-C immunoregulatory Chinese medicine for a long time for 5 years. The abdominal tumor recurred for 6 years at the time of follow-up. The condition was stable, the control did not progress, and no distant metastasis occurred. See the above Figure.

Analysis and evaluation:

This case has a huge liquid tumor of the abdominal cavity, which recurred after resection, and a huge abdominal mass. After 1 cycle of postoperative chemotherapy, the response was large, and it was not repeated.

In June 1999, he came to the specialist department XZ1+3+4 for treatment, long-term oral and external application XZ-C immunomodulatory Chinese medicine has been used for more than 5 years, and it has been 6 years at the time of follow-up. The condition has been stabilized, no distant metastasis has occurred, the tumor has not increased further, and the tumor has survived.

Case 65

Liu * * Female 34-year-old from NSW Medical record number: XXXX

Diagnosis:

Gastric non-Hodgkin's lymphoma, involving the liver

The Figure of Treatment history of gastric non-Hodgkin's lymphoma is as the following:

1999. 6.29	1999. 08.18	2000	2001	2002	2003	2004	2005
Surgery	XZ-C	XZ-C	XZ-C	XZ-C	XZ-C	XZ-C	XZ-C

XZ-C chinese medication

Medical history and treatment:

There was a sense of obstruction after eating in February 1999, which was not taken seriously.

By April, the symptoms of obstruction were more obvious, and drinking and liquid food were also obstructed.

In May, the gastroscopy was performed for cancer of the stomach body and greedy door. On June 29, a total gastrectomy was performed at Union Hospital.

The pathological section is: non-Hodgkin's lymphoma of the stomach, involving liver tissue, spleen and stomach large and small curved lymph nodes.

Due to his weakness, no chemotherapy or other treatment was done after surgery, he came to Shuguang Oncology Clinic on August 18, 1999 to take XZ-C immunoregulatory anti-cancer medicine XZ-C1+4 as an adjuvant treatment after surgery.

After taking the medicine for 2 months, the general condition is good, the spirit and appetite are good.

He has been taking XZ-C medicine every day for 3 years, and the abdominal B-ultrasound is reviewed every year, and there is no abnormality.

After November 2002, she felt that she was in good condition and her mental appetite and physical strength were good, so she changed to taking XZ-C medicine intermittently.

On January 18, 2004, when he came to the outpatient clinic for follow-up treatment, he was generally in good condition, had good mental appetite, flat, soft abdomen, unbuckled and abnormal, but the right hand was sometimes weak, but the left hand activities and grip strength were normal, and he could do housework.

The follow-up visit in April 2005, the general condition was good, no discomfort, and the patient was required to take XZ-C1+4 intermittently for a long time to consolidate the long-term effect. See Figure 65

Analysis and evaluation:

This case is gastric non-Hodgkin's lymphoma, involving liver tissue, spleen and stomach large and small curved lymph nodes. After total gastrectomy, the body was thin and weak, and no chemotherapy was performed after the operation. XZ-C1+4 was used only Adjuvant therapy of immune regulation, strengthens the body and improves immunity, improves the overall immune function, and promotes postoperative recovery of patients. After the operation, the patient insisted on taking oral XZ-C immunomodulatory adjuvant therapy daily for a long time to prevent recurrence and metastasis, thereby consolidating the long-term effect. It has been nearly 6 years for the follow-up visit.

Case 66

Mei, female, 42 years old, from Wuhan worker**
Medical record number: XXXX

Diagnosis:

Non-Hodgkin's lymphoma

The Figure of Diagnosis and treatment of non-Hodgkin's lymphoma is as the following:

2005.11	2006.8	2007	2008	2009	2010
Lump biopsy	XZ-C	XZ-C	XZ-C	XZ-C	XZ-C

Non-Hodgkin's Lymphoma   XZ-C4+2+LMS+danshen+indigo

Medical history and treatment:

In November 2005, shoulder pain, fatigue, a large swelling on the left finger, and then a swelling on both sides of the groin, about the size of an egg, no pain, no fever, weakness of the limbs, biopsy at Wuhan Fifth Hospital: non-Hodgkin's Lymphoma, B-cell origin.

Zhongnan Hospital's consultation opinion: Non-Hodgkin's lymphoma (anaplastic large cell lymphoma, cellular), immunohistochemistry:

CD32(+), ALD(++), EMA(+), CD20(+), CD799(+), CD3 (small CD43(-), CD15(-).

On August 16, 2006, due to financial difficulties, the patient did not receive radiotherapy or chemotherapy. The patient came to Shuguang Oncology Specialty Clinic for treatment on August 22, 2006. The first check-up at the outpatient clinic:

The general condition is good. There is an incision scar on the left, the crypts of the thighs on both sides are slightly full and uplifted, and the posterior buckle of the left neck and the large lymph nodes of about broad bean are treated with XZ-C4+XZ-C2+LMS+MDZ+Eshu. The patient's appetite improves, continues XZ-C2+4+chuanguong+diashent for three months, the patient feels that the physical strength is gradually recovered, and continue XZ-C2+4+Indigo Naturalis+Danshen+Glycyrrhiza for three months, the situation is obviously improved.

The patient continues to take the XZ-C series of medicines, comes to the outpatient clinic once a month for review and take medicines. It has been more than 5 years since XZ-C immunomodulation and anti-cancer Chinese medicine has been taken for a long time. The patient only takes XZ-C medication without taking Western medication and without chemotherapy. The patient came to the outpatient clinic for a follow-up visit on September 26, 2010. The general condition was good, the walking activities were as normal, there was no discomfort, the mental appetite was good, and the patient played cards every day. See the above Figure.

Analysis and evaluation:

This patient has bilateral groin masses, about the size of an egg, and a biopsy is surgically removed. It is a non-Hodgkin's malignant lymphoma with B cell origin. Due to financial difficulties, radiotherapy and chemotherapy cannot be used. He came on August 22, 2006 Shuguang Oncology Specialist Clinic uses XZ-C immunoregulation series of treatments, only XZ-C2+XZ-C4+LMS+Indigo Naturalis+danshen, without other treatments, comes to the outpatient clinic every month to get medicines, and insists on long-term medication for more than 5 years. Good health.

This example prompts:

Non-Hodgkin's malignant lymphoma can be treated with XZ-C4+1+LMS, and the drug has been used for a long time for 5 years, and XZ-C immunomodulation therapy is used only, without any radiotherapy or chemotherapy. The general condition is good, and the health condition is normal. It has a more satisfactory effect.

Case 67

Gao XX, female, 38 years old, Qinhuangdao worker
Medical record number: XXXX

Diagnosis:

Non-Hodgkin's lymphoma marginal zone cell type, recurrence after splenectomy after multi-course chemotherapy and radiotherapy

The Figure of Diagnosis and treatment of non-Hodgkin's lymphoma marginal zone cell type, recurrence after splenectomy and multi-course chemoradiation is as the following:

2002.	2000.	2000.9	2000.6	2005.	2005.3	2005.	2006.	2006.	2007.	2008	2009	2010
06	6.29	2002.01	2004.5	02	2005.5	11	04	07	01.07			
	07.10		right lung									
			infiltrating			LN large	Hilar	Chem	XZ-C	XZ-C	XZ-C	XZ-C
					splenectomy	behind	LN large					
						right ear						
	radiotherapy				splenomegaly							

250

Right neck LN 2.3cm	13 weeks chemo therapy	18 cycles Chemo		3 cycles of chemo	2 cycles of chemo	XZ-C2+LMS+MDZ+Qingzhu
Biopsy	+interferon+ CR				LN disappear	
lymphoma						
put						

Medical history and treatment:

Biopsy of right neck LNX 2.3cm in June 2030:

Follicular center cell lymphoma,

Radiotherapy from June 29 to July 10, 2000,

13 cycles of chemotherapy from September 2000 to March 2002,

From June 2002 to May 2004, the right lung was infiltrated, followed by another 18 cycles of chemotherapy. In 2005, he was found to have splenomegaly and the spleen occupied, and he underwent splenectomy.

Pathology showed:

Indolent lymphoma, small lymphocyte type,

CT: Left hilar lymph node, longitudinal wrist and axillary lymph nodes were enlarged. After 3 cycles of chemotherapy, the enlarged lymph nodes disappeared.

In November 2005, the lymph nodes behind the right ear reappeared, and he received two cycles of chemotherapy.

In April 2006, the lymph nodes behind the left neck and right ear were enlarged, and lymph node biopsy was performed. Postoperative pathology: marginal zone lymphoma, CT revealed that the posterior carina of the vena cava was under the carina, and the hilar LN increased and enlarged.

Due to consideration of non-Hodgkin's lymphoma, after splenectomy, recurrence after multi-course chemotherapy and radiotherapy, the patient comes to Shuguang Oncology Specialty Clinic on January 7, 2037 for treatment with XZ-C4+XZ-C2+LMSMDZ+ Qingzhu + Shanzi Mushroom + V it, after taking the medicine, the general condition is good, the spirit and appetite is good, and the condition is stable.

Take XZ-C immune regulation anti-cancer Chinese medicine alone as above for nearly 4 years, take the medicine daily, no more radiotherapy and chemotherapy, no symptoms Swollen lymph nodes, the condition is well controlled, and the condition has been stable and good for several years. See the above Figure.

Analysis and evaluation:

This patient is non-Hodgkin's lymphoma. After a long course of chemotherapy, XZ-C immunoregulatory Chinese medicine has been used alone since January 7, 2007. It has been more than 4 years and can stabilize the condition. The general condition is good; the patient has good appetite, no radiotherapy or chemotherapy, the patient picks up the medication every 3 months for long-term.

This case suggests:

XZ-C immune regulation and control Chinese medicine can improve the patient's immune function and prevent recurrence and metastasis.

9. **A typical case of chemotherapy + XZ-C Chinese medicine in the treatment of acute lymphoblastic leukemia**

Case 68

Zhao** Female 34-year-old Wuhan cadre
Medical record number: XXXX

Diagnosis:

Acute Lymphoblastic Leukemia

The Figure of the treatment process of acute lymphoblastic leukemia is as the following:

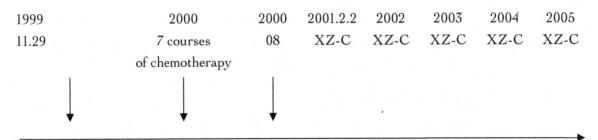

1999	2000	2000	2001.2.2	2002	2003	2004	2005
11.29	7 courses of chemotherapy	08	XZ-C	XZ-C	XZ-C	XZ-C	XZ-C

Acute lymphatic leukemia(ALL) autologous peripheral blood red blood cell stem cell transplantation

Medical history and treatment:

The patient was hospitalized in Beijing People's Hospital on November 29, 1999 due to the diagnosis of "acute lymphocytic leukemia". After 7 courses of chemotherapy, he underwent autologous peripheral blood stem cell transplantation in August 2000, but hematopoietic recovery was not satisfactory after transplantation. The blood picture of the three lines is low, WBC 0.5X109/L, PLT5X109/L, hemoglobin 46g/L, all rely on fresh blood transfusion, blood transfusion once every 8-9 days for 250mL.

During his hospitalization in Beijing, he had received 10 blood transfusions and 14 platelet transfusions (on average, once every 10 days).

He returned to Wuhan from Beijing in February 2001, and came to Shuguang Oncology Specialty Clinic on February 2 for treatment with xz-c immune-regulating traditional Chinese medicine XZ-C1+XZ-C2+XZ-C-8 to have chest protection and blood production.

In April 2001, the white blood cells, red blood cells, and platelets gradually increased, but the transfusion of fresh blood and platelets was gradually stopped, and then XZ-C immunomodulatory Chinese medicine was used completely.

The patient is persisting in taking XZ-C1+4+2 for a long time for 1 year and 7 months, the condition gradually recovered, and now the general condition is good, the complexion is ruddy, the spirit and appetite are good, talking and laughing, walking as normal, and the health condition is restored. The patient was on September 4, 2003 to go to the United States and took half a year of XZ-C Chinese medicine to the United States to continue taking it.

In 2004, the patient immigrated to Canada again, and continued to take XZ-C1+4+2 Chinese medicine for immune regulation and Shengxue Tang, mailed every 3 months. The patient called from Canada in April 2005, Generally good, good mental appetite, good sleep, working in business, no physical discomfort, good recovery. See the above picture.

Analysis and evaluation:

This patient had acute lymphocytic leukemia. After 7 courses of intensive chemotherapy, he underwent autologous peripheral blood stem cell transplantation in August 2000. The recovery after transplantation was not satisfactory. The three blood lines were low and he relied on transfusion of fresh blood and platelets. On February 2, 2001, he started taking Chinese medicines such as XZ-C1XZ--C4+XZ-C2 and Shengxue Tang. After 4 months of taking the medicine, the blood picture gradually recovered. After 1 year and 7 months, the patient's blood picture and health were obvious He has been taking the XZ-C immune-regulating and control Chinese medicine for 4 years. The patient's health has recovered well. He is engaged in commercial work and has no physical or mental discomfort. The curative effect is satisfactory.

The Experience:

Leukemia with chemotherapy + XZ-C immunomodulation Chinese medicine to protect the marrow and to produce blood and increase immunity can achieve relatively satisfactory long-term results. The essence of this disease may be immunochemotherapy. It had been 7 years since the follow-up visit, and his health was good.

Case 69

Hu** Female 64-year-old woman Xi Shu Accounting
Medical record number: XXXX

Diagnosis:

Multiple myeloma with powdery degeneration at the base of the tongue + hypothyroidism

The Figure of Diagnosis and treatment of multiple myeloma with powdery degeneration at the base of the tongue + hypothyroidism was as the following:

2007.2	2007.3-2007.6	2007.10	2008	2009	2010
Mandibular soft tissue puncture	ChemotherapyX6 times	xz-c	xz-c	xz-c	xz-c

Multiple Myolema   XZ-C4+2+ Sichuan First + Huomu + Qinggao

Medical history and treatment:

In December 2005, the mandible was swollen and the familiar sound was heavy. The examination showed that the base of the tongue was hypertrophy. After radiofrequency ablation, it became bigger again.

In December 2007, the mandibular soft tissue puncture was performed in Zhongnan Hospital. The result: mandibular muscle amyloidosis. Bone puncture results: multiple myeloma.

He received 6 cycles of chemotherapy in the Department of Hematology, Zhongnan Hospital. On October 10, 2007, he came to Shuguang Cancer Specialty Clinic for integrated Chinese and Western treatment. Outpatient examination: the general condition is good, the mentality is good, the tongue muscles are large and even the speech is not clear, and the jaw and cheeks are obvious. The swelling was hard and swelling. It was still undergoing chemotherapy at that time.

The XZ-C immune control and regulation Chinese medicine was used to protect Thymus and promote blood, improve the microcirculation, and cooperate with the treatment.

The disease is human multiple myeloma, which should be treated with anti-cancer treatment, and it should be treated with amyloidosis of the root of the tongue muscles, which should be treated to improve microcirculation, promote blood circulation, reduce fatigue, and reduce swelling and dissolution.

Three months after taking XZ-C4+XZ-C2-XZ-C3+ Limonine + Chuan Shao Jiao + Huo Shu Shi Shi Qing Zhu, the condition is stable and improved. After half a year of taking the medicine, the condition is obviously improved, the appetite is good, and the complexion is ruddy, The general condition is good. It has been nearly 4 years since the patient came to the clinic for follow-up visits and refilles medicines every 2 months. See the above picture.

Analysis and evaluation:

The patient's lower collar was swollen, and the root of the tongue was enlarged. Pathology after puncture: multiple myeloma, powdery degeneration of the lower collar muscle. On October 10, 2007, he started taking XZ-C4+2 and other immune control, blood circulation and fatigue, to improve the micro Circulating traditional Chinese medicine, the patient has been taking XZ-C Chinese medicine for a long time for 4 years, and the condition is stable and generally in good condition.

The above case tips:

1. XZ-C immunoregulatory Chinese medicine is supplemented of the treatment after radical mastectomy to assist, protect the thymus gland to promote immunity, protect the marrow to produce blood, protect the central immune system, improve the patient's overall immune function level, and help the patient to recover, and prevent Cancer recurrence and metastasis.

2. All of the above cases insisted on taking XZ-C immunoregulatory Chinese medicine for many years. After taking the medicine, they were generally in good condition, with good appetite and good long-term effect. It is to prompt: XZ-C immunomodulatory Chinese medicine is safe and effective, and no obvious side effects have been seen after long-term use.

How to evaluate the efficacy of adjuvant therapy after radical cancer surgery, it is impossible to use tumor size as an indicator, because the cancer has been removed. Good quality of life and long survival time should be used as indicators. For the cases exemplified above, XZ-C immunomodulatory adjuvant therapy has been used for more than 5-10 years after surgery, and the recovery is good.

Case 70

Peng xxx Female, 58 years old, Xianning
Medical record number: XXXX

Diagnosis:

Ovarian serous papillary cystadenocarcinoma

The Figure of the treatment process of ovarian disease is as the following:

2007. 3.15	2007.6	2008	2009	2010 12-18
Total uterus + adnexectomy	XZ-C	XZ-C	XZ-C	XZ-C

Ovaries

XZ-C1+4+5 +LMS+MDZ

Medical history and treatment:

Five years after menopause (that is, in 2005), there was no obvious cause of vaginal bleeding, the amount was small, and no treatment was given.

In the next 2 years (that is, 2007), there was no obvious cause of Mingdao bleeding in January, and the B-ultrasound at Xianning Coin Central Hospital showed: "Mixed pelvic mass".

A total uterus + bilateral appendages + appendectomy was performed on March 2007. Intraoperative findings: a large head mass in the right appendage area, cystic and solid, left ovarian atrophy, the adhesion of intestines and bilateral appendages and the pelvis wall is tight, and the large omentum envelops it.

Postoperative pathology: ovarian serous papillary cystadenocarcinoma, postoperatively due to frailty, no chemotherapy,

On May 11, 2307, she came to Shuguang Cancer Specialist Clinic to take xz-c immunomodulatory anti-cancer Chinese medicine for postoperative adjuvant treatment, with XZ-C1+5+LMS+M DZ+V it, and insisted on long-term medication for 4 years. After returning to the outpatient clinic and taking medicine, the general condition improved significantly after taking the medicine.

On July 7, 2010, the color Doppler ultrasound re-examination at the Provincial People's Hospital showed no abnormalities in the liver, spleen, pancreas, and kidneys, and no abnormal signals in the pelvic cavity. The patients were generally in good condition. See the above picture.

The Evaluation:

This patient was ovarian cancer. She did not receive chemotherapy because of his frailty after the operation. She only took XZ-C immunoregulatory anti-cancer Chinese medicine as an adjuvant treatment after the operation. She has been taking long-term medication for 4 years and has undergone a comprehensive review recently and is in good health.

This example prompts:

XZ-C immunoregulatory anti-cancer Chinese medicine can be used as an adjuvant treatment after ovarian cancer surgery.

The effect is good. Why insist on taking XZ-C immunomodulatory drugs for many years? It is because this is in line with the biological characteristics of cancer cells.

Case 71

Deng XXX, female, 61 years old, Hunan
Medical record number: XXXX

Diagnosis:

Uterine cancer, rectal cancer

The Figure of Treatment process of cases of uterine cancer and rectal cancer is as the following:

2002.12.10	2006.3,6	2007.1.21	2008	2009	2010.	12.18
Uterine surgery resection	Rectal cancer	XZ-C	XZ-C	XZ-C	XZ-C	Radical

uterus	retect					
cancer	cancer			XZ-C		

Medical history and treatment status

On December 10, 2002, it was found in Henan Cancer Hospital that squamous cell carcinoma in situ of the cervix was performed. The uterus and ovaries were removed by surgery. There was no radiotherapy or chemotherapy after the operation.

On February 15, 2006, the Xuchang Central Hospital found a moderately differentiated adenocarcinoma at 5 cm of the rectum.

On March 6, 2006, she underwent a radical resection of rectal cancer, Dixori operation, 25 postoperative radiotherapy and oral Xeloda at the Cancer Hospital of the Chinese Academy of Sciences.

From July 2006,she was given intravenous treatment in Xuchang for 4 cycles, and then thymosin was used.

Due to fatigue, fatigue, and anorexia, the patient came to Wuchang Shuguang Oncology Specialty Clinic on January 21, 2007 to use XZ-C immunoregulatory anti-cancer Chinese medicine as postoperative adjuvant treatment, and take XZ-C1+4+5+LMS+MDZ +Vit, follow up and take medicine every 3 months, has been taking medicine for 4 years, and the health condition has recovered well. See the above figure.

The Evaluation:

This patient is uterine cancer, and rectal cancer 4 years later. After surgery, the immune function is low, and radiotherapy and chemotherapy are performed, which further reduces the patient's immune function, and even becomes fatigued, fatigued, and anorexia. After long-term adherence to XZ-C immune regulation and control Anti-cancer traditional Chinese medicine has been around for 4 years, the health condition is good, and the appetite is good.

Case 72

Xu XXX, female, 43 years old: Farmer
Medical record number: XXXX

Diagnosis:

Uterine squamous cell carcinoma, stage IV

The figure of diagnosis and treatment of Uterus squmous cancer is as the following:

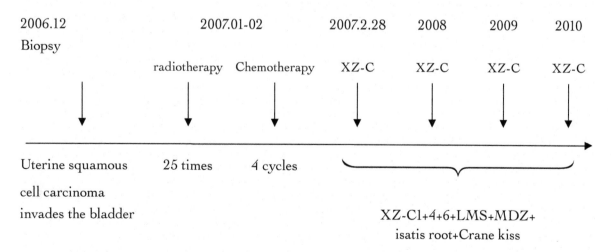

2006.12
Biopsy

2007.01-02

2007.2.28   2008   2009   2010

radiotherapy Chemotherapy   XZ-C   XZ-C   XZ-C   XZ-C

Uterine squamous

cell carcinoma

invades the bladder

25 times   4 cycles

XZ-C1+4+6+LMS+MDZ+
isatis root+Crane kiss

Medical history and treatment:

In September 2006, the vagina was bleeding for 3 months.

In December 2005, Tongji Hospital showed that the cervix was cauliflower-like, and the biopsy showed papillary squamous cell carcinoma, anemia, 25 times of radiotherapy, 4 cycles of chemotherapy, and the patient had a large response.

In December 2006, cystoscopy invaded the bladder.

On February 28, 2007, he came to Shuguang Oncology Specialty Clinic to use XZ-C immunomodulatory anti-cancer Chinese medicine treatment. Taking XZ-Cl+464-LMS+MDZ+ Banlangen+Xianheqi, long-term adherence to the medication, good general condition, good appetite, and return visits to the outpatient clinic every three months. So far, it has been nearly 4 years, and his health has recovered well.

The Evaluation:

This patient was squamous cell carcinoma of the uterus. She had already invaded the bladder at the time of discovery. She was weak and had no surgery. She received 25 radiotherapy and 4 cycles of chemotherapy. The patient was then treated with XZ-C immunomodulatory anti-cancer Chinese medicine for a long period of time. After taking the medicine for nearly 4 years, the patient's health condition has recovered well. Every three months, the patient comes to the father's clinic in Wuhan to collect medicine from the county seat, walking and moving like normal people.

POSTSCRIPT (1)

MY FATHER

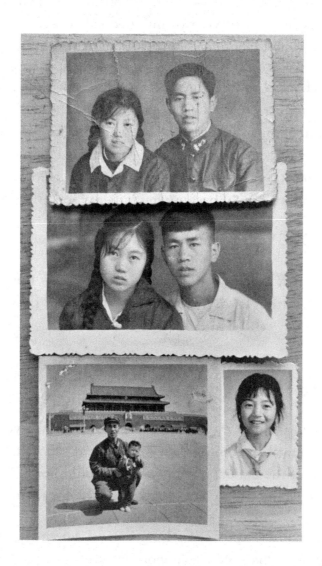

The top two pictures are my father and my mother joint picture. The picture which my father held me was taken when my father the first time saw me close to his working place after I was born. The right picture which there is only a girl is me when I was young in China.

During I wrote this book, I recalled my parents a lot, especially my father's face with wisdom and smile and confidence, which encourage me to work well and to master the skills and many times I try to get encourage and wisdom from them and try to use them to do more things for others and to live well and to live happily.

Sometimes my tears were full of both of my eyes to release my emotions for my guilt of no respect to my mother. I feel that don't have a lot of memory for my mother. I realize that I love her deeply. She was extremely beautiful and smart.

My mother was a senior OBGYN doctor in her hospital and passed away at her late 30 years while I was the second year of my medical school (at that time I was 17 year-old) and at that time I just knew a little of medical things.

During I wrote this book, I recalled my parents a lot, especially my father's face with wisdom, which encourage me to work well and to master the skills and many times my tears were full of both of my eyes to release my emotions for my guilt of no respect to my mother. My mother passed away at her very young age. I didn't have a lot of memory for my mother, only something such as when I was young, she took to go to work during her night shift duty in the hospital because my father was on the duty night.

My mother was an OBGY doctor in the different hospital with my father.

My mother passed away at her late 30 years while I was the second year of my medical school (at that time I was 17 year-old) and at that time I just knew a little of medical things.

So far I didn't know what is the exactly reason why my parents passed away, however both of they didn't have cancer.

The following many years after my mother passed away, I was very emotional about my loss and I still remembered that when my medical school teacher taught about the diseases in front of the patients, many times I could not help my tear dropping off. I know and understand deeply how hard it will be for them to lose the mother.

I was so emotional and moved by something when I saw my patients. I wish I can become a good doctor so that I can save more lives.

I missed my mother deeply and I feel deeply guilty for I didn't realize that she was very important for my future life. Here I deeply apologized to my mother. Please my mother, forgive me and forgive your daughter no respects to you.

My mother was very important for me.

Before she passed away and when I was in the medical school, she went to my school to clean all of my things during my break time and cleaned my bed and my clothes, etc. I was so spoiled by all of these at that time.

Even if I was the toppest student in my entire medical school, that my mother passed away changed my whole life.

Since then, my life went pretty difficult and extremely hard. Without my mother's protection and guide, my life is extremely difficult, especially my father's several marriages. That several unsuccessful marriages of my father after my mother passed away made my father's life hard and made my life more difficult and traumatic.

Whenever I thought of losing mother which causes the miserable, I tell myself that I must keep as healthy as I can to protect and to guide my daughter, who needs me to be around her. I pray for I can become a good doctor to save more lives and to help people to live health and to live younger without diseases.

Aging is the disease which it should be treated.

I study very hard daily to learn the new and old medical knowledge to help others and myself to live health and to live longer and to live younger. Along with the technology and science development, our human being will live close without death. Our health is controlled by ourselves. We are the driver for our health.

Of course, I had happy life before my mother passed away. Both of my parents loved me most. Both of my parents wanted to follow their careers. Every weekend my father took me to the bookstore to buy the books and almost the bookstore was the necessary place which we would come every weekend.

My family had a little library which there were full of many books.

For my father, in my opinion, he was the best doctor. I have to admit that he was well trained in some aspects for his medical career and he should be the best.

He was not only to give my life, also to save my life. He saved many patients' lives.

He was working in the China capital for the important army generals before he came back the normal hosptial. He was trained in the army hospitals. One day he told me that he worked and practiced very hard and he got many award from the army such as he could put IV into the heavy bleeding patients under darkness in the running ambulance and he got that award. He had many skills which he mastered perfectly to save the patients.

He told me many of his stories such as he studied undercover with strollight after his roommates slept in the army.

He told me how he studied while he was in the army school and he always tried to get 100% perfect, how he dedicated himself to help others. How did he get the toppest level in the field? (this is why I got 100% score on my anatomy class, I tried to remember each part in our body).

My father also is the first one who guided my idea of **fasting medicine** to treat disease many years ago which is the treasure of chinese Dao religion. He has huge knowledge in medicine.

I deeply missed my parents and appreciated them for their love and their care. During I wrote this book, I tried very hard to recall many of my parents' ideas, especially my father's words and his thinking. I always wanted to know how he saved many of the patient life during the emergency situation.

He had the knowledge on many things which are perfect for me to apply now. I was crying and crying while I found the discipline is very important to keep healthy.

He combined the religion, medicine, and social skills to save the patients' health. He is the first to tell that lifesty plays important role in our healthy such as nutrition, fasting and sleep,etc.

Chinese army medicine has the great contribution to maintain the patients' health, which was perfect.

I pray and pray for God's blessing daily.

Bin Wu

POSTSCRIPT (2)

MY MOTHER FOR MOTHER'S DAY

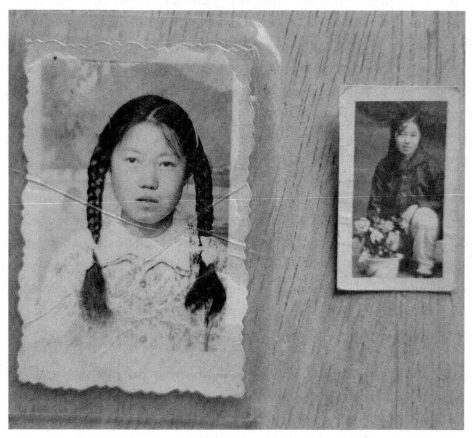

Happy Mother Day to all of the women!

I was planning to spend time in New York this weekend, however I felt extremely tired so that I decided to rest at home and to write something in order to remember my mother and hope she could forgive me of I didn't have time to think of her, to go back China and to put a punch of flower in front of her grave by my own hands. As usually, I bought a cluster of pink gerbara putting at home to express my memory for her and for the mothers and asked her for forgiveness.

After I become a mother, I realized that to become a mother is the most difficult job, especially my daughter had severe eczeme. Because my mother passed away more than twenty years, I barely remember how much love she gave me and what she looked like exactly. When I saw her pictures, I saw she had a pair of beatiful and big eyes, long and think braid, which she was very beatiful in my eyes.

I don't know how much her personalities influenced me, however a few things which I remembered will stay in my mind like crystals forever:

She brought her children alone to look for my father: she told me that once she took me, several months and my sister, one year and ten months older than me, to look for my father by taking more ten-hour train. At that time my father was a new surgeon in Army in Beijing and worked very hard and got many rewards from his work. However, he couldn't go home to see us after my mother had me. Eventually my mother decided to look for my father and wanted him to see us. On the way to look for my fahter, many people liked my sister and me and gave my mother great help. I tried very hard to imagine what it looked like. My mother loved my father very much and understood my father very much.

The naval blue color uniforms: because her children are only girls and there is no boy at home, my mother always paid attention to our appearance such as my clothes were always a little bit unique and looked very pretty such as she bought several navy dark blue uniforms including the pants, bufferfly skirt,,,,,,,,,. Many of my classmates always asked why my clothes looked perfect. My mother wanted her daughters to look good. In my homtown no matter where I went, many people would tell me that they knew both my mother and my father and respected them very much.

She cried at the station while I left my hometown for my medical college: At the station when I turned my head to wave to my mother through the window, I suddenly saw my mother starting crying and two eye red and tears flowing through her face. At that time, I was shocked and asked myself why my mother cried. I was very excited about going to my college and that was the first time I would leave my hometown alone to live outside home. In 1985 I didn't get good scores on China National Tests when I graduated from my high school, however my father put me into a medical school because I was his only hope for medicine and wanted me to study medicine and to read his and my mother's medical books, which occupied half of the rooms because he liked to buy the books. Both my mother and my father didn't send me to my college at my first trip because my mother was very busy and my father was out of town for a conference. One of my father's close friends sent me to my school and arranged everything for me in my college at that first trip. When I was the school the first week, I started cried everyday and wrote the letters everyday and called my mother everyday. I realized that I missed them very much. Soon after my father finished his meeting, both my parents came to my school and stayed with me a few days. One of my family's close friends, a surgeon, was the president in the affiliate hospital of the medical college. He let others arrange everything for my family while my parents were my college at the first time. Thanks God, in my medical school I studied very hard and had many number scores in all of my classmates. I spent eight years there.

"Why didnot you sleep?" I asked my mother: Many times I woke up during the midnight, I saw my mother still sat there. " Mon, what time is it and why didn't you sleep?", I asked her. " I am waiting for your father." I don't understand why my mother loved my father very much like this way. My father had a habit which was to go back the hospital to talk with the patients and others in the evening after his dinner, espically for the complicated surgery patients. He concentrated on his skills very much, however my mother always took more care of us and her family.

She told my father that she felt guilty because she didn't give his boy to carry his family name: when my mothe was very sick, one day in front of me she told my father that after her death she hoped me not to stop my father to marry again because she felt guilt that she didn't have a boy for my father. I was very upset about her words even if now. My tears were in my eyes and couldn't say anything. I didn't understand why my mother loved my father like this way and considered everything for my father. My mother passed away at her early some fourty years old and I was in the third year of my medical school. After my mother passed away, my father did married several times, which hurt me deeply. I don't know the names of the women who my father was married with again and again because I didn't want to know and never talked with anyone of them.

She was sent to the countryside to work by her hospital for one year: when I was in the first grade of my elementary school, my mother was sent to work in the countryside for one year by her hospital several hours away from my hometown, my father took care of us alone. I didn't know what happened until before I graduated from my college to choose my specialty. My father wanted me to pick up an easy specialty and didn't be involved in many responsbilities and had a comfortable life. At that time my father briefly mentioned the reasons why my mother was sent to the countryside for one year because one patient was heavily bleeding in the delivery room,,,,,. My mother was the OBG doctor for that patient. He told me that in the hospital sometimes it would be very difficult to decide what were wrong and what were right so that the doctors should learn how to protect themselves from any unnecessary things while they took good care of their patients.

She always took more responsibilties for us such as she took me to go to work with her during the night: When I was young, many times my mother took me with her to work and slept in the duty room because my parents didn't work in the same hospital and both of them were on-call at the same times. My mother supported my father's career very much and wanted him to be excellent and perfect on his duties. She never complained of anything in front of her children. I didn't understand why my mother did many things like this way.

She picked me up home from my college school when I finished my second medical scholl in the summer in 1987, which was the last time she went to my school: I was very spoiled by my mother and never did any chores while she was with me. In 1987 after I finished my second year medical school, my mother came to my school and help me cleaning my bed and my apartment and everything. At that year I didn't get good scores on a small subject and told my mother that I didn't like my teacher on that subject. My mother told me that please don't say anything bad about my teachers,,,,,.. I didn't listen to her at all at that time,,,,. Mon, please forgive me now and please forgive me not respect you which I should. Not until you passed away, I didn't realize that you were very important for me and how much love you gave me. I just got and got from you. Mom, did you remember? When you were dying in the hospital, I told you that I felt very scared about everything. Now I feel that I was very selfish and didn't understand my mother at all. Mom, please forgive me and forgive my unmaturity.

I didn't remember how much love I gave my mother before, which I pray for her forgiveness. Mother, would you please forgive me about anything which I didn't listen to you?

Bin Wu

REFERENCE

1. <<Walked out of the new road to conquer cancer>>.

Author: Xu Ze, Bin Wu, etc. Published by Authorhouse Inc.
(Including the eight books : Volume I, II, III, IV,V,VI,VII,VIII) from 2018 to 2019

2. <<The road to overcome cancer>>. Authors: Xu Ze, Bin Wu, etc. Published by
    Authorhouse press. In 2016

3. <<The new progress in cancer treatment>>. Authors: Xu Ze, Bin Wu, etc.
    Published by Authorhouse press. In 2018

4. << On innovation of Treatment of Cancer: Cancer immune treatment combined
    Chinese with Western medicine>>. Authors: Xu Ze, Bin Wu, etc. Published by
    Authorhouse press. In 2015

5. << New concept and new way of treatment of cancer>>

Author: Xu Ze, etc. Translator: Bin Wu, etc. Published by Authorhouse press. In
2013.

6. << New concept and new way of treatment of cancer metastasis>>

Author: Xu Ze, Bin Wu, etc. Published by Authorhouse press. In 2016

7. <<Condense Wisdom and Conquer Cancer for the Benefit of Mankind >>
    (including two books: Volume I, II)

Author: Xu Ze, Bin Wu, etc. Published by Authorhouse press. In 2017

**All of the above books are published by Authorhouse and can be found in
Authorhouse.com**

Printed in the United States
by Baker & Taylor Publisher Services